'I highly recommend this important
experiencing an epidemic of tiredness
Lisa's succinct description) is a significant cause of depression, fear
and anxiety. Rest and release can be wonderful supports. Lisa skilfully
offers practical options, guiding the reader through the problems and
the possibilities.'

— *Norman Blair, Senior Yin Yoga Teacher, Teacher Mentor and
author of* Brightening Our Inner Skies

'Finally, a book and a method that apply the wisdom and practices
of yoga and therapeutic principles to the widespread issues of
sleeplessness! Those who suffer from insomnia can find true relief
using this approach.'

— *Anodea Judith, PhD, bestselling author of* Wheels of life,
Eastern Body-Western Mind *and* Chakra Yoga

'Lisa has written her life work and generously shared it for the benefit
of all. Born of her own interest and need to understand and experience
deep, restful sleep, and the obstacles that prevent it, Lisa integrates
ancient and modern wisdom in a practical guide to sleep. From
yoga asana to neuroanatomy, Lisa distills for the reader the lessons
of science and self-care in manner that is useful for psychotherapists,
counsellors and yoga therapists seeking to integrate mind, breath and
body approaches to help themselves and their clients experience the
restorative benefits of sleep.'

— *Lisa Kaley-Isley, PhD, E-RYT-500, C-IAYT; Founder, Life Tree Yoga
with Lisa; Director, The Yoga Therapy Clinic; and Board of Directors,
Yogacampus Yoga Therapy Diploma Course*

'This book is a gift for the yoga teacher, healer or therapist who wants
to help others to rest better, especially for those working with pregnant
ladies or new mothers. This approach brings in what others forget —
that we are spiritual and soulful at our very core, and that healing and
wellness must integrate this essential part of ourselves. I love the idea
at the heart of this book: that sleeplessness can call us to awaken.'

— *Erika Tourell, Senior Yoga Teacher,
Teacher Trainer, Doula and Mother*

'A must for people who suffer from insomnia. Sanfilippo demonstrates a profound knowledge of yoga and sleep disorders, clearly explaining postures and breathing techniques.'

— *Dagmar Härle, Master of Psychotraumatology, RYT, TCTSY Facilitator, Somatic Experiencing Practitioner*

'Lisa brings in-depth knowledge and experience to this thorough and accessible work. Jam-packed with practical techniques and helpful understanding, this book will support those looking to get their sleep back on track and gain much-needed energy.'

— *Jillian Lavender and Michael Miller, Co-Founders, London Meditation Centre/NY Meditation Center*

'This manual on sleep, insomnia and an approach to helping clients tackle their sleep disturbances is clear, well researched and practical. It is an invaluable resource for clinicians dealing with sleep disturbances and is a good stepping-stone for helping medical professionals to approach sleep problems in an embodied manner. Lisa Sanfilippo incorporates an intuitive sense about the body with well-evidenced therapeutic and scientific knowledge.'

— *Dr Shivanthi Sathanandan, MBBS, Consultant Psychiatrist, Camden and Islington Foundation Trust and National Health Service Practitioner Health Programme UK*

Yoga Therapy for Insomnia and Sleep Recovery

of related interest

Yoga Therapy as a Creative Response to Pain
Matthew J. Taylor
Foreword by John Kepner
ISBN 978 1 84819 356 7
eISBN 978 0 85701 315 6

Sleep Better with Natural Therapies
A Comprehensive Guide to Overcoming Insomnia,
Moving Sleep Cycles and Preventing Jet Lag
Peter Smith
ISBN 978 1 84819 182 2
eISBN 978 0 85701 140 4

Principles and Themes in Yoga Therapy
An Introduction to Integrative Mind/Body Yoga Therapeutics
James Foulkes
Illustrated by Simon Barkworth
Foreword by Mikhail Kogan, MD
ISBN 978 1 84819 248 5
eISBN 978 0 85701 194 7

Trauma-Sensitive Yoga
Dagmar Härle
Foreword by David Emerson
ISBN 978 1 84819 346 8
eISBN 978 0 85701 301 9

Yoga Therapy for Fear
Treating Anxiety, Depression and Rage with the Vagus Nerve and Other Techniques
Beth Spindler
ISBN 978 1 84819 374 1
eISBN 978 0 85701 331 6

YOGA THERAPY
FOR INSOMNIA
AND
SLEEP RECOVERY

*An Integrated Approach to Supporting
Healthy Sleep and Sustaining Energy All Day*

LISA SANFILIPPO

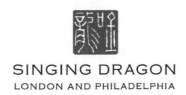

SINGING DRAGON
LONDON AND PHILADELPHIA

First published in 2019
by Singing Dragon
an imprint of Jessica Kingsley Publishers
73 Collier Street
London N1 9BE, UK
and
400 Market Street, Suite 400
Philadelphia, PA 19106, USA

www.singingdragon.com

Library of Congress Cataloging in Publication Data
A CIP catalog record for this book is available from the Library of Congress

British Library Cataloguing in Publication Data
A CIP catalogue record for this book is available from the British Library

ISBN 978 1 84819 391 8
eISBN 978 0 85701 348 4

Printed and bound in Great Britain

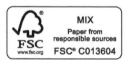

MIX
Paper from
responsible sources
FSC® C013604

This book is dedicated to the memories of two very special people who will always reside in my heart and visit me in my dreams, Kevin Collis and Susan Z. Watson.

Contents

Acknowledgements

Massive thanks go to the Sanfilippo family – Margaret, Charles and Diane, the late Barbara and Bill, and the yogis of the family: John, Bob and Susan, for introducing me to tofu and gurus, malas and mantras. And my expat family: Simon Austin, Beverly Bonner, Susanne Miller, Jane de Teliga, Grace Saunders and Katinka Blackford Newman. I am also eternally grateful to Anodea Judith, who showed me a model for yoga therapy that resonated with my heart and stirred my soul's calling.

I also wish to acknowledge an excellent group of commentators and reviewers, including Katy Baldock, Dr Shivanthi Sathanandan, Dr Matteo Bernardotto, Kate Hewett Taylor and Theo Kyriakos. A special team of people commented on trauma and trauma-sensitive yoga, including Alexandra Cat, Frances Ross, Linda Karle and Theodora Wildcroft. Very special thanks to Heather Mason of the Minded Institute for her collaboration and contributions. Others whose inspiring teaching and care contributed to this book include Jono Condous, Jillian Lavender and Michael Miller, and Dr Barbara Mariposa. With thanks to Masha Pimas for her attentive and lovingly created drawings and to Jonathan Thompson for modelling some of the practices.

I consider myself incredibly lucky to have the unflagging support of my two London yoga homes, where the workshops and courses were born. I am ever grateful to Jonathan Sattin and his team at Triyoga, and Elizabeth Stanley and her team at The Life Centre and Yogacampus. My gratitude and appreciation also go to each person who has allowed me to offer them support in bringing their sleep back to balance. We have learnt from each other.

Thank you as well to the incredibly patient team at Singing Dragon: Sarah Hamlin, Victoria Peters and Vera Sugar.

And finally, warmest hugs to places and friends who offered me homes in which to write, soothing cups of tea and fresh air: Lucilla Green and her Casa Verde in Ibiza, Anais Theyskens and Sivaroshan Sahathevan, Hopewell and Lantern Cottages and the Hundred Monkeys in Glastonbury.

Disclaimer

Every effort has been made to ensure that the information contained in this book is correct, but it should not in any way be substituted for medical advice. Readers should always consult a qualified medical practitioner before adopting any complementary or alternative therapies. Neither the author nor the publisher takes responsibility for any consequences of any decision made as a result of the information contained in this book.

Introduction to Sleep Recovery

A Yoga Therapy Approach

Overcoming Insomnia and Finding Better, More Restful Sleep

Sleep is a vital resource: it restores and replenishes us on every level. For increasing numbers of people today, sleep has become elusive or problematic. Maybe insomnia has become more prevalent or maybe we are talking about sleep problems more openly than ever before. Either way, sleeplessness or poor quality sleep can stem from – or contribute to – a whole host of other imbalances in our health or mental health. When we can't get to sleep, sleep restlessly, wake in the middle of the night or stumble out of bed after what should be a full night's sleep feeling groggy and unrefreshed, this can create a vicious cycle of difficulties with everything from memory to mood, upsetting hormones and brain chemistry.

This book is written primarily for therapists – manual/body therapists and psychotherapists, doctors, teachers, healers, helpers and clinicians of all kinds. People come to us seeking solutions and we want to help them get out of pain, get back into balance, and start enjoying their lives again. If your client or patient knew what to do to solve her problems, *and* could take action, she wouldn't be coming to you. You will have some responses that relate to your own training and experience. In this book you will find a holistic approach and a set of powerful tools to approach better sleep which may add to these. The five-layered approach in this book seeks to address the whole person with creative, flexible solutions. When taken together and used sensitively and skilfully, they can help your client to recover their sleep in the short and long term.

Trouble Sleeping? Insomnia and Beyond

We seem to exist in a tired-but-wired society. We need remedies that help us get to sleep at bedtime and to feel awake during the day, respecting our bodies and their natural rhythms. The British physician Dr Jim Horne spent a professional lifetime working with insomnia and sleep problems in clinical medical practice, and wrote two books on the topic (Horne, 2007, 2016). He found that *the best medicine for good sleep is to have a happy, healthy life.* Although we hail from different training and experience, I agree with Dr Horne! When we are happy and healthy, of course we tend to sleep well at night.

As Dr Horne found, the limitation of modern medicine is that it needs to focus on treating acute problems, rather than maintaining wellness – and happiness is, in a way, out of its territory. A yoga therapy approach takes as its task the full range: dealing with the effects of acute problems, resolving the underlying issue by repairing the imbalances that created the problems, and restoring and maintaining wellness throughout the life cycle. It even goes further – promoting not only physical wellness but also a more profound attunement to one's mental, emotional and even spiritual aspects. **Through a yoga therapy approach, insomnia can, in a sense, be a path to awakening.**

In this book, we'll look at more conventional approaches to insomnia, including the medical models, and then explore the resources offered through a holistic yoga therapy approach. Many of the options offered here are wholly consistent with the medical research and evidence, especially where they intersect with cognitive behavioural approaches. Other parts of this programme extend far past the domain of modern medicine, bringing in time-tested yoga-based traditional methods, which put power back in the hands of the person to balance and heal herself before problems resurface.

Insomnia and Sleep Problems: What Are They and How Many People Are Affected?

We'll start practically – with the question: what does it mean to have *good* sleep? Good sleep means that we wake feeling refreshed enough to get through our days with enough energy to meet reasonable daily demands. The amount of sleep needed varies from person to person within a range from roughly seven to nine hours per night. Some people sleep more or less, with more or less disturbance in their sleep, without it being problematic. On the other hand, good sleep does not mean that a person puts their body in the bed, shuts their eyes, immediately falls into a deep sleep, never stirs and emerges refreshed after exactly eight hours every night. Good sleep doesn't mean that the human body has endless energy when awake. Nor does it mean that we can over-ride our need for rest and down-time in addition to sleep. **We are not machines that switch from 'on' to 'off' and back on again with constant energy levels all day.** We have ebbs, flows and rhythms. Most of us have variations in sleep across a week, and our sleep is affected by many factors from food and drink to light exposure or our emotional state. We'll deal with many of these factors in the coming chapters in some detail, and a range of excellent books take many of these discussions even further than we can within the scope of this yoga therapy book.

Even given normal fluctuations, sleeplessness has become a world-wide problem. The rates of insomnia are thought to be roughly similar in the US, UK, Germany, Australia and Japan (Havens *et al.*, 2017), with some studies showing 10 to 20 per cent of the general US population experiencing insomnia, 50 per cent of whom experience chronic insomnia (Buysse, 2013). Some studies put the figure in the US up as high as 23.6 per cent (Roth *et al.*, 2011). In one recent British commercial survey (Dreams, 2016), more than 60 per cent of respondents said they were unhappy with the amount of sleep they were getting, almost 30 per cent said they never wake up feeling refreshed, and 74 per cent of their respondents said they actively worried about not getting a good night's sleep. Another 2017 study (Sleep Council, 2017) reported that almost one third of Britons (30%) felt that they slept poorly.

This is not only a *personal* health problem, but also a *public* health issue. Insomnia can cause lost productivity at work and greater risk of road traffic and machinery accidents, and can lead to misjudgements in providing needed care for others. Insomnia can indirectly increase health care expenses borne by individuals, public health systems or insurance providers through impairing immune system functioning, and through possible links to heightened cancer rates and increased anxiety and depression. **Repairing broken sleep before it reaches a critical level and helping people to overcome insomnia can make a tremendous contribution to our individual and collective wellbeing.**

So, let's look at insomnia from a clinical perspective. Clinicians call insomnia *chronic* when a person has difficulty sleeping for three months or more, and at least three times per week, despite the person having the opportunity to sleep enough – not because of shift work, travel, etc. – and that it causes 'clinically significant distress': the person is hindered in some way in personal/family life, work or other important areas. This may involve sleepiness, fatigue, problems with low mood, irritability, or difficulty thinking or trouble remembering things.

Some sources divide chronic insomnia into primary insomnia, where the insomnia appears to stand alone as a problem, and secondary insomnia, in which there's an identifiable underlying cause, for example when a psychological or medical condition, a medication or drug misuse is involved. In practice, I don't encounter much insomnia that has occurred for absolutely no reason at all.

My fellow yogi and researcher Dr Sat Bir Khalsa and I co-wrote a chapter for a yoga therapy book (Mason and Birch, 2018). Dr Khalsa notes that although reasons for insomnia can be genetic, environmental, behavioural, psychological and physiological, these all contribute to psychophysiological hyper-arousal (Buysse, 2013). In other words, insomnia is usually brought about by *something*: a stressful event, a trip involving jetlag, a prescription medication that interferes with sleep quality, hormonal changes, parenting crises, a trauma being re-triggered, or the build-up of bad sleep habits in conjunction with one of these or other inciting incidents.

Put simply – there are lots of things that make us keyed up and too wired to sleep properly. And, to make it worse, when we don't sleep well, we can start acting or thinking in ways that we think will be helpful but actually harm our sleep.

Here are some common examples, as my co-author Sat Bir Khalsa pointed out in our chapter on yoga therapy for insomnia cited above:

- We might spend extra time in bed trying to 'catch up' on sleep, but this starts to break the body clock's sleep–wake time mechanisms.

- We might pay more attention to sleep: 'try to sleep' or 'worry about sleep' – which backfires because the worry about sleep itself sparks up our nervous systems into hyper-arousal, which of course perpetuates the insomnia.

- We might try to do things (work, watch movies, use social media, etc.) right before bed to try to make ourselves tired or distract from the distress of 'maybe I won't fall asleep', but the lack of wind-down time in itself can lead to poorer quality sleep.

- Using substances like caffeine or other stimulants to wake up and alcohol to fall asleep can backfire, making it harder to sleep and feel awake.

- Taking naps may remove the 'sleep drive' needed to have a good *night's* sleep at the right time, much like having a snack can dissipate the hunger for a full meal.

So even when the initial problem is long-gone, the habits used to try to manage the initial insomnia may actually sabotage sleep even further.

The yoga therapy for sleep recovery programme in this book helps people to manage sleep disturbances before they become intractable insomnia or if it *has* become entrenched long term. We'll look at how to recover and restore good sleep naturally and sustainably. You'll learn a range of strategies that take down the level of actual physiological arousal in the body that prevents sleep (wired-ness), help to combat tiredness at the wrong times of day for sleep, and take away the 'I won't be able to function' worry that often adds insult to injury when it comes to insomnia. Clearly, insomnia and sleeplessness are multi-layered problems that require multi-layered solutions.

Physician, Heal Thyself

No other health problem seems so pervasive as sleeplessness – so much so that many people have come to view habitual poor sleep and daytime sleepiness as normal, and regularly resort to stimulants to stay awake during the day. I attended a recent conference on Sleep Medicine at the Royal Society of Medicine in London, held in an auditorium with no natural light, and noted that several participants dozed off during the presentations, to be pepped back up with tea and coffee in the break. The structures of our working environments often lack acknowledgement of the human needs for light, rest and exercise, and we seem to be paying the price in terms of our sleep–wake patterns, dozing off and being prodded awake with stimulants.

It has become clear that we need effective, sustainable sleep support at the ready. The tools in this book help our clients to 'meet life on life's terms': we can help them to respond to life's demands for energy and activity as well as sleep and rest with the resources that support both, sustainably. With our help, they can overcome insomnia, find better rest and meet each day more alert, alive and awake.

You will be able to offer something to each person that enables them to combat interrupted sleep, hyper-alert nervous systems, physical tension, emotional turmoil and many other conditions to repair lifelong sleep problems or to prevent the insomnia reaching damaging levels without the use of medication.

It's Not Just Mind Over Matter

While 'top-down' or 'mind over matter' methods of sleep support assume that the mind can somehow switch off the body, this seems only partly effective. Human beings have evolved over millions of years, with the more recent, highly powerful thought-centre of the neocortex as only one part of our processing system. We are also structured in a way that enables bodies to quickly and powerfully influence our brains, responding to cues about safety. The state of tension or relaxation in our muscles and in our breathing sends powerful signals to our brains, and neurochemistry follows, altering the global condition of our system. Instead of trying to simply change your thoughts, the yoga therapy approach enables you to change your body, your breath, your thoughts, emotions and trust in the natural capacity for restorative sleep – without a 'command and control' approach that treats us like machines to be switched on and off.

What you learn in this book works *with* the complex fabric of the human being – beyond simply body and mind. Instead we look at how we function in terms of **five levels called koshas or sheaths**. This gives us insight into finer ways to identify and correct imbalances in the whole person.

We also acknowledge that each person has a unique constitution: a physical and mental nature. Some may even acknowledge a 'soul nature'. In this, people with different natures will tend towards different types of sleep imbalances, and will respond to the types of remedies and practices that bring them back into balance appropriately for their 'type'. We draw upon Ayurvedic classifications that typify human beings in terms of the elements found in nature, and their characteristics, as a way to exemplify these differences. These elemental types are referred to as **Ayurvedic doshas**, or **doshic types**.

When we have trouble sleeping, we need to relearn some aspect of our patterns and habits to restore ourselves to health. If sleeplessness has become entrenched, unravelling these patterns may take time but the results will be sustainable. While people suffering from insomnia or disrupted sleep patterns can come to rely on any number of external things (pills, potions, scents) or special accessories of all sorts, quick fixes are often expensive, become ineffective the more you use them, or are unsustainable in other ways.

For example, sleeping pills may act quickly and provide a quick fix, but their help may come at a cost. When they work initially, they can become ineffective when used regularly over time (Hauri and Linde 1996), they can inhibit the mental-rest-related REM (Rapid Eye Movement) sleep, or in the case of Zolpidem (commonly referred to as Ambien) studies show that it works without dependency, but that a range of strange adverse effects can result: 'sleep-related complex behaviours' like sleep eating or even sleep driving, parasomnias, amnesias, hallucinations and even suicidality, at much higher rates compared to all other drugs (Wong *et al.*, 2016, 2017).

When the external things a person relies upon to sleep are not available, the sleep-compromised person is likely to panic, setting in motion sleep-sabotaging anxiety. The approach in this book instead teaches sustainable self-support so that you have everything you need to slow down, sleep better, and feel rested and alert throughout the day. Your clients will not need to rely on expensive equipment and props – they will build the innate capacity to relax and restore from the inside out. For this reason, we don't focus on externally guided meditations, and all that I offer can be learnt in person, or from a book or video, practised (which is *essential*) and then easily remembered with minimal external prompting.

Unlike sleeping pills or tablets, yoga practices and the self-care habits in this programme become *more* effective the more you use them. The stretching postures help the body to become more relaxed, more adaptive, and less tense physically. Simple breathing techniques (pranayama) make your breathing easier, deeper and freer all day, giving better access to states of relaxation more quickly and easily. Meditation helps to create a relaxed yet aware state of mind without panic or tension, making it easier to calm a ruminating mind before bed or upon awakening in the middle of the night.

If they use these techniques, our clients will no longer need us for the same problems or issues again and again. I am thrilled when my students and clients no longer 'need' me and they *graduate* from their yoga therapy for insomnia classes or consultations. Do all of my graduates zonk out every night at the same time and sleep eight hours, bouncing out of bed the next morning, every morning? No. Because they are not machines. Their bodies' needs and ability to rest will fluctuate with life changes day to day, much like many people experience fluctuations in appetite for food. However, when my clients follow the guidelines and use the practices in this programme, they experience a dramatic, irrevocable and positive change in quality and duration of sleep and rest, and know how to calm themselves into a state of rest when needed. They experience the benefits in terms of their personal habits and quality of life.

- In this book you'll learn to assess sleep problems from a holistic perspective. Your vision will include multiple aspects of a person's experience and how these affect their sleep, and what they can do differently.

- You'll round out your set of tools and approaches, or learn where to signpost on to other qualified practitioners, to help your clients truly overcome sleep problems.

- Step-by-step instructions help you to experience each practice yourself and, where you're qualified (and insured!) to do so, to pass these practices on to your clients whether one to one or in groups.

A Personal Story

I have a tall shelf full of books about sleep and overcoming insomnia. Many have been written by professionals with a great deal of useful information from many angles. However, they seem to be written by people who either haven't ever had chronic debilitating insomnia, or won't admit to having had it! For some it's a speciality area because it's academically interesting or a 'career choice'. This was not the case for me. I began researching holistic approaches to recover from my own devastating insomnia nearly 20 years ago. I *needed* a way to heal myself. I had visited my doctor, and after a brief examination was told there was nothing physiological causing my insomnia, but that at my age (early twenties at the time), the doctor was disinclined to prescribe medication to sedate me as she knew it would not truly solve the problem. She offered me the best advice I could have been given: that I should consider learning yoga and relaxation techniques including meditation, and if the insomnia persisted, to explore psychotherapy. I did all of the things she suggested, and used my sleeplessness as a wake-up call. I knew I didn't want to be sick and tired for the whole of my adult life, so something drastic needed to change.

In the late 1990s Ambien was new on the sleep-drug scene, and cognitive behavioural therapy (CBT) for insomnia was not widely available. This was also long before countless yoga sequences were available on YouTube. In fact, yoga was not nearly mainstream, and neither YouTube nor the variety of wonderful online yoga instruction channels existed. Back then, the only information I could find on 'yoga for insomnia' was a passing mention in the B.K.S. Iyengar classic book *Light on Yoga* (1995). His prescription totalled five lines of bullet-pointed text. By contrast, what you find in this book includes two decades of trial and error, training in Anusara yoga, investigations into the therapeutic applications of yoga, exploration of traditional Ayurvedic approaches, a fruitful collaboration with the research-based yoga therapy training organization The Minded Institute, and more than a half dozen years of training and practice in transpersonal psychotherapy at the Centre for Counselling and Psychotherapy Education in London.

In the time since I overcame my own chronic insomnia, the pace of living seems to have accelerated, with the inception not only of ubiquitous mobile phones, but a complete online revolution and a smartphone in nearly every hand. I began and ended a career in public policy while starting to teach yoga, and heard from more and more of my students during this time that they were having trouble sleeping. I began offering workshops, courses and private sessions over the years, sharing what had worked for me, devouring every book and approach I could find. This enabled me to keep improving my own relationship with sleep while helping others. I was fortunate in that the two most established and well-respected yoga studios in Europe – Triyoga and The Life Centre – supported this work and gave me space and time to develop the programmes I offered. I've since gone from being the *only* yoga specialist offering workshops that focus on sleep problems to being simply the first of many to do so. I have trained other teachers and health practitioners, and incorporated more knowledge through the years of tailoring the approach to fit many types of people. The research and clinical experience began with my own story, and now draw upon the stories of countless others, with plentiful thanks to many individuals and institutions. These are, I hope, all mentioned in the dedication and gratitude pages.

Sleeplessness as a Wake-Up Call

I shared my personal story with you, because if we look more deeply, conquering insomnia may not just be about fixing a particular problem but an opportunity to come back into balance, as I did, with even greater health and wellness than before. Not being able to sleep can be a wake-up call. For me, and for many of my clients and students, it has created a call to awaken. As healers and practitioners of health and wellbeing, we can see more deeply to both solve the problem at hand and create the opportunity for our clients to become more healthy and whole in all of life. I'll show you how you can use these holistic maps, approaches and practices to understand and help heal insomnia, enabling your clients and patients to sleep better tonight and for the rest of their lives.

Real People, Real Examples

Look carefully at the examples of real people (whose identities and personal details have been changed to protect their anonymity) in this chapter and throughout the book. You'll see different body types and psychological makeup, life challenges and resources (physical, psychological and emotional). Each person has her own tendencies and blind-spots or gaps. Some would never-in-a-million-years-do-yoga, while others were die-hard yoga fans before they came to yoga to recover their sleep. While there are common sleep saboteurs and sleep saviours, these are different for each individual. This programme teaches you to work with common principles and to tailor for different constitutions.

For all of the people who are mentioned in this book as examples, though their needs and personalities were very different, there are common features:

- They were all sick of sleeping poorly or not at all.

- They wanted to heal.

- They took responsibility for their own health, with my help.

- They did the work, and when they couldn't or weren't willing to, they owned up to it and we adjusted their practices.

Assessment

The tools and processes in this programme and in this book *work*. But only if you 'work' them. They need to be used and put into action. So the first step is to assess a client's level of frustration and pain, and whether this is motivating the person to change. When tailoring the approach to each person, it's vital to fit in the changes and practices with what they're already doing, and make changes over time. This is why I most often have a client see me for six sessions, and take them through the layers in this book week by week, adding and adjusting skills, tools and practices to meet their needs.

Why Not Just Yoga, and Why Yoga Therapy?

By the time some people reach me, non-yoga people may be so desperate to sleep better that they will 'try anything' even if they think that yoga means 'unicorns and rainbows'. They have lost faith – almost – but not completely. They may have tried sleeping pills, CBT, special supplements, pillow sprays, new beds and a range of other attempts to solve the problem. Others may never have considered that they could stop feeling frustrated and exhausted.

Other people may be 'into yoga' but have not learned or successfully used yoga to find consistent better sleep. I teach in the two biggest yoga studios in London, which employ many expert teachers of modern yoga styles. Many of my students and clients already practise yoga that has not yet helped them, in itself, to overcome insomnia and sleep problems.

Today, what is called 'yoga' may involve intense workouts ranging from the slow and steady Hatha or Scaravelli to classical Primary Series Ashatanga, Power Yoga, Vinyasa Yoga, Rocket Yoga and Hot Yoga. It's become increasingly common to practise yoga postures and do breath work to dance or pop music, with has a high beat-per-minute pace that entrains the heart rate to follow suit. While these styles of yoga have benefits in terms of body conditioning and concentration, they are often too fast or muscular to let the nervous system settle. In addition, some modern yoga studios and gyms offer intense and stimulating classes late into the night, when most people with sensitive sleep need to begin 'amping down'. These may create a sense of immediate tiredness when the 'workout' is over, but may not work to train the nervous system to rest deeply. To support our sleep, there is no substitute for the quieter side of physical yoga – following the breath, ability to regulate one's own heart rate, and work with innate natural rhythms.

While beneficial in their own ways, most modern styles of yoga practice may not properly teach the essential relaxation skills needed to sleep better. Given that we are in the midst of a poor-sleep epidemic, the yoga teaching community would better serve the public by learning how to support (and not to sabotage) sleep as a key aspect of wellbeing.

A Yoga Therapy Approach

While yoga is traditionally a practice geared toward enlightenment, transcendence or spiritual awakening, yoga therapy uses many of the tools of yoga for more day-to-day purposes: alleviating specific physical and mental disorders. Yoga therapy utilizes both yoga-based and physiological or medical assessments in order to create a programme of treatment. According to the International Association of Yoga Therapists (IAYT), 'Yoga therapy is the process of empowering individuals to progress toward improved health and well-being through the application of the teachings and practices of Yoga.' I particularly like a definition given by the late Georg Feuerstein PhD I found on the IAYT web site:

> Yoga therapy…integrate[s] traditional yogic concepts and techniques with Western medical and psychological knowledge. Whereas traditional Yoga is primarily concerned with personal transcendence on the part of a 'normal' or healthy individual, Yoga therapy aims at the holistic treatment of various kinds of psychological or somatic dysfunctions ranging from back problems to emotional distress. Both approaches, however, share an understanding of the human being as an integrated body–mind system, which can function optimally only when there is a state of dynamic balance. (Feuerstein, n.d.)

To help place our work in context, I introduce four clients from my practice: their sleep problems and how a holistic approach based in yoga ideas and techniques helped them. Most people who land in my classes or in my consulting room have tried other approaches or therapies before coming to me. We'll see how they overcame insomnia and experienced this process as a foundation for fuller health and wellness.

First we review some of the tools of yoga according to the eight-limbed approach most commonly found in yoga training today. Then we look at one holistic way of seeing people – as having five layers or koshas, an idea that comes from yoga's Upanishads. We will then meet several of my clients (whose names and identifying details have been changed, of course) who have different personality and physical 'types' as understood through an Ayurvedic lens, and see how the perspective and practices of yoga addressed their sleep problems.

Table I.1: The Frameworks Involved in Yoga
Therapy for Insomnia and Sleep Recovery

Framework	How it's used in this programme	Source
The Eight Limbs of Yoga	This is a framework for understanding yoga practices which includes: ways of relating to oneself, orienting ethically towards others, use of posture(s), breathing that directs prana (life force), inward focus away from external sense information, and cultivating a meditative state for the purpose of enlightenment.	Attributed to Patanjali, in a traditional text called the Yoga Sutras, which is referred to in many yoga teacher training programmes in the West.
The Five Koshas or Layers	Offers a map for understanding people: as made up of layers. Disturbances in sleep can occur for physical, energetic, mental or emotional reasons. These are used for assessment, and the programme uses practices from the eight limbs of yoga, and other healing modalities, to bring balance back to each layer.	The Upanishads, a yoga philosophical treatise, which offers an understanding of the nature of the human being.
The Seven Chakras	A way of understanding the 'energy system' of a human being which recognizes correspondences between physiological, energetic and psychospiritual characteristics of embodiment and offers a way to redirect energy (balance, increase, decrease) for healing or transcendent purposes.	Described as subtle energetic centres in Tantric yogic texts, modern interpretations posit correlations between these energetic centres and anatomical structures, psychological attributes and developmental stages.
The Three Primary Doshas or 'Types'	A way of understanding a person's physical constitution and personality. A person will often have one predominant 'type' and the other two in some proportion will balance out their constitution.	Ayurveda: a system of traditional healing and wellness that developed alongside yoga.

The Eight Limbs: Classical Yoga Practices

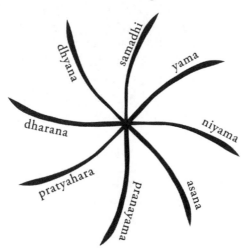

The Eight Limbs of Yoga in the Yoga Sutras of Patanjali

While yoga texts are diverse in origins and mostly focused on spiritual development, the modern approach to yoga teacher training has seized upon the Yoga Sutras as a shared text. While not intended as a therapy approach initially, but as a path to transcendence, the eight limbs of yoga spelled out in the text, and modified with modern understanding, can be of great value when adapted for therapeutic purposes.

An integrated approach to yoga for better sleep offers valuable practices of yoga postures (asana), breathing and energy management (pranayama) and meditation. However, yoga therapy also seeks the integration of our whole being so that we are not only sleeping better – and alleviating the symptoms of dis-ease – but also moving towards becoming fully 'awake' as human beings. The yogic texts and technologies point in the direction of enlightenment – which is often aptly called 'awakening'.

Modern yogis have seized upon the process outlined in the second pada (part or, more literally, foot) of Patanjali's Yoga Sutras (Shearer, 2002). While classical yoga was geared towards 'transcendence' – rising above daily embodied experience towards enlightenment – our yoga therapy approach is rather different. Yoga therapy puts to use yoga tools and understandings to meet worldly challenges with peace, equanimity, adaptivity and grace. Philosophically speaking, this is a Tantric notion – that of transcendence or enlightenment in 'immanence' or being-in-the-world. In this way, the body is not a problem to solve or a burden to offload. It is seen as sacred. This integral body-positive, multi-limbed approach alters the familiar constructs adapted from the Yoga Sutras. Thus, it's a living tradition applicable to the householder's experience and a framework for holistic healing ('householder' is used as a term that contrasts with the yogi as an ascentic or religious devotee). The sections below explain the relationship of the eight limbs to our yoga therapy for insomnia approach.

Yamas and niyamas: how we make choices and take action in our lives. The yamas are about our relationship to the world of others in society, the outer environment, or nature. These aspects of life can signal areas of harmony or disharmony – and disharmony may lead to disruption in natural balances including sleep. The niyamas discuss relationship with oneself internally – keeping one's own mental and emotional balance through a balanced lifestyle. These in particular relate to the physical aspects of sleep, and taken generally can offer a framework for good life-hygiene as well as sleep stewardship.

Asana: physical postures (seat). The yoga asana sequences offered in this programme create relaxation and alertness as needed in the physical structure of the body, as a container for consciousness.

Pranayama: breath practices (direction of prana or energy). The breath and self-acupressure practices in particular, as well as the asana, direct prana and subtle energy towards the balancing and grounding needed for better sleep, or the alertness needed for the waking state.

Pratyahara: retraction of the senses/disengagement. If we are in the sense-world, attention is turned outward. In our overly sense-stimulated society, slower, mindful yoga practices including meditation and internally focused asana and pranayama teach us to disengage from the outer world and turn within.

Dharana: focus/steadiness of mind (container). If the mind is continually harangued by external impressions or constant pre-occupation with thought, it is difficult to sleep. The training of meditation and release of emotional tension are essential to allowing us the steadiness and calm, expansive focus needed for sleep.

Dhyana: meditation. Classically, this limb of yoga pertains to the mind merging with an object that contains it, leading to an experience of connection and oneness. Something special happens to us when we feel we are part of nature, the universe or life force. We start to de-centre our concerns, pains and worries, and begin feeling a sense of humour, joy or peace.

Samadhi: equanimity consciousness. The deepest peace that is reached can equate to a sense of surrendered slumber.

The Five Koshas:[1] A Layered Map

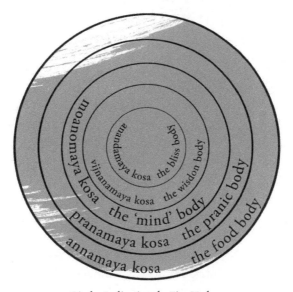

Circles Indicating the Five Koshas

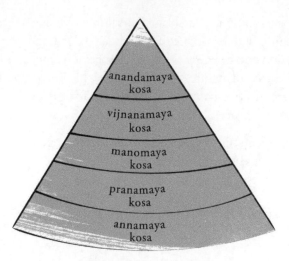

The Five Koshas Pyramid

In this sleep recovery programme, we draw upon a framework called the panchakosha, or five sheaths, a map of *embodied consciousness* derived from a traditional text called the Upanishads (Feuerstein, 2011).[2] I make no claims to this being true to the traditional expression of each of the koshas. In fact, I have adapted them liberally, for contemporary therapeutic purposes, as have some of my colleagues (Koay, 2012; Stiles, 2010, 2013). The sections in this book are organized according to the five layers as I have distinguished them for this yoga therapy for insomnia task, which may be constructed differently from the way my colleagues have done. I also outline the layers in conjunction with the practices outlined in the eight classical limbs of yoga, and incorporate modern adaptations and additions from other traditions where I have found them helpful in practice. As the Upanishads and Yoga Sutras were not originally intending to offer a yoga therapy model in laying out the five koshas and the eight limbs, we are all using these concepts for different purposes from those intended. Arguably, although not historical, they are useful.

Using a map doesn't show you the territory itself but it does guide you on your journey. Viewing people as made up of five layers lets us address more than just body and mind, and provides a more detailed map so that we come to 'read' people with more subtlety and offer practices that build balance in each layer. Based on your professional

---

2   For a more in-depth discussion of the koshas see http://hareesh.org/ blog/2015/12/16/the-five-koshas-and-the-five-layered-self-a-comparison.

training and personal interests, you will have more knowledge or background in one or more areas.

To help people sleep better, I start with the outer-most, physical layer and move more deeply as the work progresses. For multi-week group courses, I address one layer per week and teach the practices and habits that relate to physical, energetic, mental, emotional and soulful aspects of balancing our sleep. It is much the same in working with clients one to one, but I can shift the emphasis to focus on the layer or aspect of the self that is most imbalanced. When I work with people individually over a longer time period, an awareness of the seven-chakra system, which will be discussed later in the book, helps me to work with the deeper-seated dimensions of a person's sleep problem. If you take the image of a tree, you can see the tree-rings radiating outward horizontally as the five koshas, and the structure from roots to treetop as embodying the root-to-crown journey of the seven chakras.

The Physical Body

The yoga tradition calls the outermost layer – our physical bodies – the 'food body'. This includes muscle, bone, organs, tissue and even blood and body fluids. This encompasses the dense physical structures that have weight. What we eat and how we relate to the outer environment and the physical body are included here.

Physical yoga practices support sleep by calming the body and preparing it for rest at night. Other practices induce a sensation of wakefulness and alertness appropriate to the time of day. These are all tailored in support of circadian rhythms. Daily practice and habit guidelines integrate physical keys to sleeping better by managing habits throughout the day to 'sleep proof' your day.

Sleep-inducing poses.[3] Particularly in yoga therapy for insomnia, clients will learn and practise yoga postures (asana) to pull tension out of the muscles, and to signal relaxation from body to brain, creating feelings of relaxation, calm and safety. Physical tension is interpreted by the brain as 'I'm not safe and therefore shouldn't relax'. Getting the safety signal from the body to the mind can start with pulling tension out of the key muscles and expanding essential areas that the brain uses to interpret pre-cognitive cues.

---

3   The terms 'poses' and 'postures' are used interchangeably throughout the book.

Table I.2: The Five Koshas as Adapted in this Yoga Therapy for Insomnia and Sleep Recovery Programme

Kosha with definition	Aspects addressed by this part of the approach	Yoga practices	Examples of therapies and interventions	Key perspective for recovery
Annamaya kosha: the physical body	Physical tension, physical imbalances and the stress response, sleep hygiene, habits of food, drink, exercise, circadian rhythms.	Simple Sleep Sequence: Calming and grounding. Restorative Poses: Reconditioning the nervous system and reinstating the relaxation response. Wake-Up Sequences: Creating alertness without harmful stimulants.	Osteopathy; chiropractic; nutritional therapy; deep tissue/fascia release such as rolfing; Feldenkreis; Alexander Technique; sleep restriction techniques; medication/psychiatry; dietary approaches from the medical through to traditional holistic including Ayurveda and Traditional Chinese Medicine/Five Elements.	Where do I store tension and how can I release it so that my body doesn't signal 'alert' or tension? Habits of what we ingest and do can contribute to poor sleep (saboteurs) or to good sleep (saviours).
Pranamaya kosha: the energy body	Changes to breathing directly affects the nervous system towards stimulation or relaxation. Circulation. Energy levels/exhaustion and agitation. This layer bridges the physical and mental aspects of the nervous system.	Pranayama: Three-part breath to stretch the body from inside. Altering length of inhale vs. exhale creates different effects. Breath practices create the relaxation response, or create alertness. Marma points for self-acupressure affect the circulation and nerve responses throughout the body.	Energy: Reiki; acupuncture; acupressure in the Eastern systems; marma therapy. Breath: CPAP machines;[1] therapies to improve breathing.	How can I breathe to manage my stress or make myself feel more alert? How can I come out of continual stress responses?

kosha			
Manomaya kosha: the mind body	Inability to 'switch off' the mind. Anxiety about sleep. Misperceptions about sleep.	Self-guided techniques: Meditation actually alters brain wave patterns and can 'process' thoughts before they flood in at bedtime. Thought logs/ journalling are useful tools here as well.	Psychiatry and some psychotherapies such as cognitive behavioural therapy; mindfulness techniques; psychoanalysis; other guided mindfulness or yoga nidra work with the mind and other layers.	Thoughts need a 'place to go'. We must work through preoccupations, clarify misinformation, de-catastrophize sleep and other anxieties. Sleep is comprised of different brain wave states. We can practise the ones that help us get to sleep and stay asleep.
Vijnanamaya kosha: emotions/ wisdom	Emotional management. Emotional stress response, ability to 'let go' and trust in sleep. Matters of conscience. Awareness of underlying trauma as a result of overwhelm, active at other levels but addressed here for our purposes.	Emotional awareness and release practices that are similar to meditation. Relationship to self and others, in the life-guidance of the yoga tradition, can foster harmony and emotional balance.	Trauma awareness processing and release work such as EMDR; TRE,[2] and Somatic Experiencing. Some psychotherapy and counselling; creative imagination, dream work, emotional freedom technique, hypnotherapy.	Difficult emotions can cause physical tension and agitation in the nervous system. They need space and processes to be worked through so that their hold can be released.
Anandamaya kosha: the bliss body/ spiritual level	What makes you feel 'awake' and how to heed the 'wake-up call' of not sleeping well. Symptoms are symbols of something we need more deeply.	Trust. Yoga's philosophical precepts orient us towards meaningful, well-aligned life and a trust in nature, natural forces, or a 'power greater than the individual effort'.	Spiritual practices; religious orientation, perspective or sense of one's place in the universe.	Living with an over-inflated sense of responsibility and lack of trust in nature can create long-standing inability to feel at home in the body and in sleep.

1   Continuous positive airway pressure (CPAP) machines help people to breathe at night when they are asleep. They are available through medical professionals and are common sleep aids for people with sleep apnoea.

2   Eye Movement Desensitization and Reprocessing (EMDR) and Tension & Trauma Release Exercises (TRE) are two modern methods of trauma release. EMDR works with the movement of the eyes as a way to unlock trauma, and TRE involves physical (shaking) exercises. Both rely on an understanding of the body and brain's mechanisms for storing and releasing trauma.

Wake-up poses. During the daytime hours, yoga postures that send 'activation' or alertness cues from the body to the brain are used.

Restorative poses. During the afternoon 'slump' that many experience in line with circadian rhythms, this approach utilizes restorative yoga postures to 'layer in rest' and 'put energy back on the grid' instead of 'borrowing from the energy credit card'.

The Energy Body

The 'energy' body is a concept that encompasses the nervous system, breath and circulation. It indicates the relationship between how we breathe and how we feel, and the importance of the message-relaying system of nerve communication between the body and the brain.

Pranayama, or yoga's breath practices, are essential tools for recovery from sleep problems and insomnia. The approach taken in this programme is gentle, emphasizing three key capacities:

- **Breath awareness** is a pathway to interoception. The breath-based body-sensation practice strengthens capacity for full and rhythmic breathing, and increases one's ability to feel and dissipate tension in the belly, ribcage, chest and shoulder areas.

- **Breath can create a state of calm.** We offer practices that stimulate the parasympathetic (rest-and-digest) part of the nervous system, appropriate for managing anxiety, stress responses and pre-sleep tension.

- **Breath can foster alertness without agitation.** Gentle breath practices stimulate the sympathetic nervous system (alertness, without the extreme side of 'fight or flight'). These bring clarity and alertness without over-agitating, and do not keep you awake as caffeine does.

Self-acupressure accesses muscle and nerve responses, and can be practised in conjunction with gentle breath work. For insomnia and better sleep, self-acupressure/marma therapy includes stimulating specific points on the hands, face and back of the neck.

The Mind Body

In the third layer we work with the mind and thoughts. Anxiety, worries and preoccupations about our lives – especially fear of not sleeping well or enough – can cause sleeplessness. Many people complain about an inability to 'switch off' their minds. Therein lies one of the primary problems – we are not machines that switch on and off. Managing heightened mental activity at night before bed or when sleep is interrupted is possible when we manage the mind, and work *with* it throughout the day. From a yoga perspective, self-guided practices act to balance and prepare the mind for sleep. We address the most common mind-over-matter approaches to sleep, so that we understand how this programme incorporates some of their best features, while bringing in additional resources.

Meditation. We use simple focusing meditation practised regularly. This builds the capacity to be awake without directed thought, and to 'drop in' to less-excited brain wave patterns more easily.

Writing. The process of slowing down the mind to the pace at which thoughts can be written by hand is a powerful practice. Many of my clients find that if they write down their ruminations, or write down the thoughts they find turning over in their minds before bed, they are able to get to sleep more easily and effectively.

Emotions/Wisdom

In this programme, we view this layer as the emotions sitting beneath the processes of rational thought, which provide a different kind of wisdom. When one's inner wisdom or emotional state is disturbed, either by not allowing 'shadow' emotions like fear, anger, sadness and grief or through being consumed with them, balance is elusive. It is at this deeper-than-cognitive level that overwhelming, frightening and traumatic experiences can retain a hold on us, long past the time when our rational minds believe us to be affected. The practices for supporting sleep at this layer address the vital role of allowing emotions to arise and be felt, processed and released.

In this yoga approach we value the role of talking therapies, referring onward where necessary, and offering some techniques to assist.

The Emotional Release Technique for those without trauma symptoms. While not a meditation in the sense described in the section above ('The Mind Layer'), this technique allows the student to sit quietly, feeling tension in the body and identifying emotions and feelings that relate. Breathing with awareness of the emotion builds the capacity to sit with it, allow it to arise, get bigger, and then fall away. This is a powerful technique, especially after removing the majority of physical tension in the body through yoga stretches.

Trauma is a term used to describe the impact of overwhelming and terrifying experiences that leave traces on our responses, long after the original events. Chapter 4 will help you to understand when post-trauma reactions may be at the heart of sleep difficulties, and offers a preliminary exploration of things you will need to consider if you're working with a person who has a post-traumatic form of insomnia.

The Bliss Body/Spiritual Level

Not sleeping well can be a profound wake-up call, with the desire to stop suffering igniting an intention to heal, and with the ability to become quiet and listen providing us with valuable information about how to do so. If we work through painful or uncomfortable experiences like insomnia, and gather the tools to come back into balance, we can emerge healthier, even happier and more attuned to our needs, on every level, than ever before. Instead of a problem-solution quick fix, yoga therapy invites us to see our health and wellbeing as sacred, and to look after ourselves lovingly. Wellness is not just the absence of suffering. In this part of the programme, we learn to listen more deeply to all aspects of the self and respond with care instead of criticism, resources instead of resistance.

In Chapter 5, I bring in the **seven-chakra approach** primarily to relate the yoga therapy for insomnia approach to the development of the individual, which I use predominantly in a one-to-one yoga therapy approach, and this is offered for those who are familiar with the model and wish to integrate their knowledge or to explore further.

Sleep Recovery

My approach to yoga therapy for insomnia encourages us to see ourselves as multi-layered individuals, and prompts us to look at aspects of body, energy, mind, heart and soul as each has a role in our health, balance and wellbeing. In addition, each person has a particular constitution in each of these layers. While there are many traditional methods of understanding people's constitutions, we'll look here at the Ayurvedic approach to understanding our 'nature'.

The Three Ayurvedic Doshas: Physical and Psychological Constitution

When we offer practices to address the different aspects of a person's problems with sleep, we also need to take into account the individual's constitution: their nature. I encourage my clients to think of our need to sleep like our appetite for food. Some people have a regular, steady appetite and all other things being equal would eat pretty much the same amount each day. Others eat more some days, less on other days, depending on their mood and habits. Others still may have disordered eating affected by body image. Emotional upset or travel can affect our appetite and digestion, much like these same factors can affect our sleep. Some of us expect normal fluctuations and accept these as part of our day to day and adapt accordingly. We all have different constitutions, and much like appetite varies by person and day to day, our sleep can do the same.

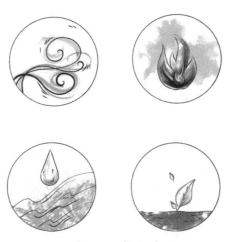

The Ayurvedic Doshas

Yoga's 'sister science', a form of traditional medicine called Ayurveda, outlines three main body–mind types. It can be useful to understand how a person's nature and relationship with external nature affect their sleep tendencies. Contemporary yoga therapy approaches may tailor the practices and habits for clients depending upon their constitution and nature (Stiles, 2010). This section draws heavily upon the work of Vasant Lad, one of the foremost authorities on Ayurveda in the modern world, and I've brought in information from his *Textbook of Ayurveda: A Complete Guide to Clinical Assessment* (Volume 2) (2007).

Through the lens of Ayurveda, we all tend to exhibit characteristics that align with different elements in nature. The doshic (constitutional) types (called in Sanskrit, 'prakruti') are determined by observation, questioning and touch: they form a general tendency in a person's physical, energetic, mental and emotional nature. Each person has some of each prakruti, in greater or lesser measure. While most often one of the constitutional aspects dominates, for some people two types are equally dominant, with the third in lesser proportion, and relatively infrequently, all three aspects may be equally dominant.

We can create balance or imbalance in our natural constitution by our actions and habits. In Ayurvedic thinking, if your present state is the same as your constitution, then you are in good balance and healthy. Diet, lifestyle, emotions, age and environment affect one's current state (for which the Sanskrit word 'vikruti' is used), in real time. Healing brings back the balance towards the individual's innate constitution.

While insomnia is generally spoken of as a 'vata disorder' involving nervousness, anxiety, ungroundedness, hyper-sensitivity, excess thought and worry (Frawley, 2000), for people with each predominant doshic type, insomnia can surface in different ways. This section discusses how imbalance for each of the prakruti/doshic types relates to sleep difficulties. With an understanding of a person's basic type, practices can be tailored to 'meet' a person in their predominant element to help to bring balance to their current state and build better sleep.

Vata (Air)

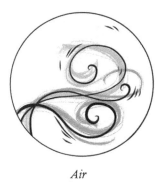

Air

Those who tend to have difficulty falling asleep and staying asleep, or wake many times during the night, may tend towards vata disturbance. Anxiety can be a symptom of a vata imbalance, and when a person has suffered trauma their nervous system can respond by exhibiting vata tendencies. People with vata constitutions tend to have light sleep and need more practices that are focused on pulling energy, prana or circulation downward in the body out of the head and into the pelvis, legs and feet. Warming practices, warming foods and grounding practices are healthy and balancing for vata types.

According to Dr Lad

Vata [has the qualities that are] mobile, cold and clear. A vata person tosses and turns in his bed, putting the head on the pillow with no sleep at all. That kind of tossing, turning and restlessness is vata insomnia. It is difficult to enter into sleep and there is continued interrupted sleep. When vata people do not get enough sleep they become dizzy and drowsy. Vata insomnia creates constipation, anxiety and fear.

A vata person often has scanty, interrupted sleep. They find it difficult to enter into sleep because their mind is active. It is difficult for a vata person to sleep in darkness because darkness is a vast, spacy thing and vata people sometimes imagine weird figures and become frightened due to their inherent fear of darkness. They often prefer to sleep with a dim light turned on. Vata sleep is variable, light and interrupted by frequent waking.

Too much vata leads to a lack of sleep. To create sound sleep we need the slow, heavy, tamasic qualities of kapha. Because of increased vata dosha, there are more of the light and mobile qualities so the mind and senses are overly alert and active.

Pitta (Fire)

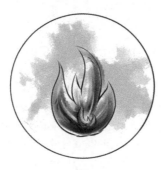

Fire

Those who have trouble getting to sleep because they are doing too much, and wake with high levels of cortisol in their system early in the morning, may tend towards pitta imbalance. They tend towards short sleep. The emotions associated with this type tend towards anger, unresolved emotions or frustration. People with a predominant pitta type may need to expend their energy and discharge it before they can attain relaxation. They may also need to balance the exhaustion that comes from 'firing on all cylinders'. Practices that balance adrenal over-exertion and that focus on nourishing the kidneys can be especially beneficial. Think of 'cooling and soothing' practices.

According to Dr Lad

Pitta people can have such incredible energy at midnight that they cannot drop off to sleep. They often like to read books at this time for this reason and unless their eyes become tired, they find it hard to fall asleep. They may read a couple of chapters and then, when their eyes become tired, fall asleep with the book on their chest; that is typical of a pitta. A pitta person cannot sleep with the light on because their eyes are bright from intense pitta in their eyes. Pitta sleep is moderate in duration but sound…

Alpa nidra is a condition of pitta imbalance – scanty sleep due to an over abundance of heating qualities, but not total insomnia as may be seen in vata-based disorders insomnia…

In pitta insomnia, there is also often difficulty entering sleep. However, once a pitta person falls asleep, he will usually wake only once generally during the pitta time from midnight to 2am. However, pitta sleep may be disturbed by small noises, even the sound of a watch ticking. When a pitta person does not get adequate sleep, he becomes irritable, critical and angry and gets burning eyes. He will criticise his bed, his light and start judging his clock.

Kapha (Water/Earth)

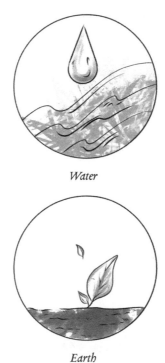

Water

Earth

Those with a more kapha constitution may be grounded naturally and tend towards lethargy. They may not get the activation they need to inspire the relaxation needed for deep sleep. More movement, sweat-inducing activity and cardio-vascular activity can be very helpful at the right times of day. Those with more kapha type of constitution may also fall more easily into depressive states. For kapha types, there may be problems with sleeping many hours and still not feeling rested: feeling groggy and tired regardless of long sleep are signs of kapha imbalance. Activating practices in the morning like Breath of Joy and Sun Salutations, kapalabhati breath (a pumping and invigorating practice often used in Kundalini yoga) and concentrating less on grounding and more on 'elevating' practices can be very valuable for people with this constitution. Energizing practices may be used in the morning and afternoon.

According to Dr Lad

A **kapha** person's sleep is heavy and prolonged. A kapha person can fall asleep right away whether there is a bed or not. They can sleep on a rug, in an alley or sitting in a chair, because they love to sleep.

Meet Some Sleepy People

The stories of my yoga therapy clients help to bring to life the principles of yoga therapy for sleep recovery, and I've changed their names and the details of their identities, out of respect for their privacy. We will return to them throughout the book, bringing in examples that relate to the different aspects of yoga therapy and how they are used in practice. Theirs are stories of exploration, increasing self-knowledge, agency and healing. Working with each of them has taught me a great deal and informed my approach. I offer them thanks, and I enjoy sharing their stories – it's an honour to see people restored to wellness and feeling more positive about their lives.

BRIAN

Brian came to me when he was regularly getting three hours of sleep a night. He had a handsome face, and with his tall thin frame, he resembled a zombie with hollow eye sockets. He seemed 'wired' and fitted the description of the Ayurvedic vata type very well. As an author, he had an active intellect and imagination. His mind could work at warp speed, and often did just at the times he should have been sleeping. Although a successful published author and university lecturer, his life felt unmanageable and chaotic due to sleeplessness. One small drama at work could set him into intense anxiety. Brian had used marijuana regularly over several years to slow his thoughts and encourage his body to relax. Running gave him respite from his over-active mind and at times exhausted him enough to sleep later in the night, but it didn't lead to longer sleep. He and his long-term girlfriend kept separate flats as he was afraid she would leave him if she were aware of the extent of his tortured sleep and self-medicating.

We began with the Simple Sleep Sequence of yoga postures for a week, reviewed in Week Two, and then progressed to some of the Deeper Sleep Sequence poses later. These helped to soften the tense, wired and jangled quality of his body. His breath was freer and longer. When doing the poses, his body settled towards the floor and he seemed broader, with improved circulation in his limbs and face.

I taught him restorative yoga poses which he was able to settle into after four weeks doing the Simple Sleep Sequence. (An earlier attempt, before doing yoga postures regularly, left him twitching, unable to relax.) He used restorative yoga poses to take a break from writing without caffeine and without creating a boom–bust stress–energy rollercoaster.

After six weeks of yoga practice, he was able to move on to meditation, which he credits with dramatic changes in his life. I ran into him on a train about five years after his last appointment with me, and I could barely recognize him. His face looked healthy and vibrant. He was not only sleeping well, but was also planning his honeymoon. We'll see Brian again later.

CATHY

Cathy is a retired Italian grandmother who came to my six-week course in London having practised gentle yoga for most of her adult life. She enjoyed yoga as a way to lessen her depression by moving her body. Though she had the long sleeping patterns of a kapha type, she rarely felt rested. She would stay up late, not feeling sleepy enough to drop off, but would sleep for up to ten hours, waking up groggy in the late morning, with little energetic spark.

Doing the Simple Sleep Sequence every night and the wake-up poses each morning helped her to create a routine, something that she lacked in retirement. The course information about circadian rhythms, about the effects of caffeine and strategies for managing difficult emotions helped her to structure her days towards better physical and emotional balance, helping her to get better sleep at night.

Cathy loved the group class: she met others of all ages and found she was not alone in her insomnia. Although her doctors were compassionate, tackling her sleep problems medically with little success left her feeling pathological, isolated and ashamed of her sleeplessness. The group setting helped her to overcome feelings of shame and strangeness, and much of her sleep-anxiety dissolved. She felt like an active participant in a social gathering: she enjoyed feeding back on her progress each week, asking questions, and getting support and suggestions for refinement.

She used the sleep log, keeping track of nights when she did the Simple Sleep Sequence and breath practices, and when she didn't. Some nights, she began to feel sleepy at an acceptable bedtime and skipped the pre-sleep yoga, but noticed that she was more apt to wake in the middle of the night or sleep more fitfully. She realized that doing bedtime yoga not only helped her to get to sleep when she needed it but also helped her to sleep more deeply and soundly, waking more refreshed in the morning. She added some morning stretches and did the Breath of Joy each day. Her kids noticed how much more energetic Cathy was in playing with her grandchildren, much to her delight. We will hear more about Cathy in Chapter 3, and learn how she used journalling to support better sleep.

SIMON

Simon was in his early fifties, a married father of two children and a high-level business consultant heavily involved in local politics. He is funny and sharp, and speaks in rapid-fire sentences, with intensity and humour. He is a natural leader, with the natural 'fire' of his pitta constitution, also fuelled by a powerful history of family hardship. His face held a lot of tension and he would sit on the edge of his seat. He came in with a notebook and reported back all his 'bad nights'. There was scarcely a pause between his sentences.

When he started my six-week group course, Simon would sleep poorly six nights out of seven each week. He struggled to fall asleep and would wake with a start in the middle of the night, unable to get back to sleep. After 25 years of success in business and politics, he began having panic attacks about both. He was vehemently not-a-yoga-person but gave my course a try out of sheer desperation, at the behest of a trusted fitness teacher he'd worked with over many years.

After the first week's session, he reported back with utter shock – he'd practised the postures each night as directed. They had made him feel less tense before bed and he'd slept noticeably better. Over the six weeks we refined his breathing to make it less forceful and smoother. We reviewed the stretches, and added some for the middle of the night if he woke up and needed help to settle back to sleep.

His sleep improved dramatically and his confidence and trust in the process had grown during the course, to the point where he wanted to explore the other 'layers' of his sleep problems in greater depth one to one.

We began with a thorough assessment of his physical habits, then nervous system patterning, managing stress and life transition issues. He asked: 'Do I have to give up wine and coffee forever?' My reply: 'If it's causing sleep problems, then if you want to sleep better it has to go, even if just for now.' When he stopped drinking coffee and switched to tea before 11am he noticed a marked difference. He also began to track that middle-of-the-night sleep disturbances were far more likely after even a single glass of wine at night. He was convinced he needed to change some long-held habits.

He kept up the foundation of yoga poses each night, and I assessed how he was doing the poses periodically to be sure he took enough time with each pose, slowed down his breathing, and completed each exhale smoothly. This was initially very difficult for him, but as he began to breathe more slowly, he felt profound changes. We began to work on how he could be present in his meetings differently – breathing more, staying connected to his body, living with less adrenaline-fuelled energy, and with more sustainable energy. Breathing more calmly throughout the day helped him to lower his level of hyper-arousal overall, which meant less tension in the day and fewer middle-of-the-night wake-ups.

For Simon, meditation became an easy 'bedrock' practice. We framed it as 'taking a meeting with himself' or 'executive-personal-time'. He decided to practise meditation in his car before entering the office, or go directly to his bedroom after work before coming down to meet his family for dinner. This helped him to 'process' his busy day and turned his night-time stream of thoughts from a torrent to a trickle. In the past, thoughts of business, family and politics would take over when he put his body in bed; now, he began giving himself time to work through these thoughts earlier in the day, leaving calmer headspace before bed.

While the benefits were real after a few weeks of yoga poses, Simon stayed with the process and has made dramatic changes in his life. He enters the room more calmly, sits back with ease, and looks less intense. He still laughs easily – and more heartily than ever.

LINA

Though her insomnia was nearly paralysing, Lina could not bring herself to attend a group yoga class or course. In groups, she would feel nervous and tense amongst other people lying down on a yoga mat. If her body relaxed a little bit, it would convulse and tighten up in a spasm, which was embarrassing and counterproductive for her.

Lina used alcohol most nights of the week to help her get to sleep because she suffered nightmares so frightful that sleep itself became a fearful prospect. In our initial meeting, she didn't want to commit to the full six sessions of one-to-one work, as she had tried so many expensive solutions that had not worked for her over many years. She wanted to see how she felt about sessions a few at a time. In the end we worked together for eight weeks.

In her case I made an exception to my requirement that students commit upfront to a course of sessions because it seemed clinically important – in the case of complex trauma, it's essential to have good boundaries and explain the clinical or recovery significance of each aspect of why we work as we do, but never to coerce or impose. It was essential that Lina was already in a well-established process of psychotherapy so that she could bring her experiences back into her therapy. Even though I am a trained therapist, to keep the boundaries clear we focused on 'just the yoga'. Sticking to what we're asked underscores the client's ability to guide her own recovery and maintain boundaries safely.

I taught her the Simple Sleep Sequence, and swapped in some poses from the Deeper Sleep Sequence where the originally offered ones looked 'triggering' or not-for-her. I allowed her to choose from the options, with no explanation needed. She enjoyed the poses, and could feel them releasing tension from her limbs. If we stayed in a stretch too long, her body would convulse and she would tighten up again. For Lina, it was a process of releasing 'enough but not too much' to create relaxation – and slowly so that her body and mind could trust the release process.

We also addressed Lina's fear of being wrecked by exhaustion following a difficult night's sleep. Three or four wake-up poses each morning became part of her routine, and she found this tremendously energizing and comforting. Instead of relying solely on caffeine, which would wake her up, but frazzle her already tired nervous system, the stretches gave her something enjoyable to help her into her body.

A few sessions into our work, Lina mentioned her 'restless legs' at night and how tense they felt during the day. The Simple Sleep Sequence's thigh and hamstring stretches helped her become more aware of how tense these muscles were all day. We added a custom-designed series of achilles, hamstring, hip and thigh stretches as well as practices to ground her feet, which she used at work to dispel tension throughout the day. I also made her aware that research shows that smoking is a risk factor for restless leg syndrome (RLS), and she tapered her intake down to vaping once per day in the morning.

In this way, we worked within Lina's window of tolerance, and helped her to manage her tension levels throughout the day so that they would not build up to unmanageable levels at night.

If I were working with Lina as her sole therapist over the long term, we might do some Somatic Experiencing work and dream work to help her to work through the content and symbolism of her nightmares, investigating what her unconscious is trying to resolve in her life. For therapists working in this way, creating the foundation of bodily safety can provide a resource.

Lina's sleep improved, and she had a greater sense of agency over her life. While she still suffered from nightmares, the quality and duration of her sleep and feelings of restful calm increased throughout our work together. We'll explore some important considerations for post-traumatic insomnia in Chapter 4.

OTHER SLEEPY PEOPLE WHO WILL SHOW UP THROUGHOUT OUR TOUR OF SLEEP RECOVERY

Silvia had had trouble sleeping since she entered peri-menopause, for which she had become reliant on sleeping tablets. She was finally able to build the confidence to come off the tablets, using the Simple Sleep Sequence and relaxing breathing techniques to take down her temperature and tension. She became better able to manage her hot flushes, mood swings and daytime tiredness by recharging with restorative poses.

Thom, a young musician working in my local cafe, shared his insomnia with me while making my decaf Flat White. I shared with him tips for managing his daily habits for better sleep.

Marielle recently came through a round of cancer treatment. Although she had always slept well before her illness, the upheaval and trauma of illness and surgery led to fractured and fearful sleep. She regained her capacity to sleep well using the techniques in this programme.

Paul found his sleep in tatters after a bitter divorce and his temper began to flare as a result. He used the tools for physical, mental and emotional sleep recovery: working through tension and weathering the difficult transitions that underpinned his inability to sleep. He used new-found resources to move through his anger to find greater perspective, balance and a regular good night's sleep.

Under the Strangest of Circumstances

Recently, I taught the Simple Sleep Sequence to a TV presenter for a programme about sleep and health. The presenter doesn't identify with having insomnia but says she normally wakes up once or more during the night to use the toilet. She did the Simple Sleep Sequence, three-part breathing and a few minutes of Little Bridge Pose in front of a TV crew with all the interruptions common in filming. Although we stopped and started, and finished the yoga practice at about 5pm, many hours before bedtime, she reported back the next day that she had slept through the night for the first time in months. A somewhat incredulous 'thank you' email arrived the next day: 'I wouldn't have believed the impact of such simple stretches and the effect of the breathing – if I hadn't experienced it for myself!'

And Now You: Practice as Resource

One premise of the Yoga Therapy for Insomnia and Sleep Recovery approach is that we bridge the gap between practitioner and client. A clinical approach views the client or patient as presenting with pathology and the clinician as providing the solution from a rational evidence-based perspective, based on randomized controlled trials and established medical protocols. This is useful and helps to ensure validity of medical approaches, but if we are to take a yoga-based, holistic approach, there is another way of knowing that is accessible to us: embodied experience.

Let's look at an extreme example: if you are healthy, you would not take chemotherapy in order to empathize with your patients undergoing cancer treatment. If you don't experience sleeplessness it would be farcical for you to take sleeping pills to understand your patient's or client's world. That would be detrimental to your health and you wouldn't really understand their world anyway.

However, with the practices in this book, even if you don't have trouble sleeping, you can *feel* the effects of the poses in your own body. They will benefit you even if they are not being used to overcome insomnia. You can experience the way your mind shifts when you do the breathing practices, and you can experience the impact of the self-acupressure points. If you do them following my guidance, they will create a sensation. They will affect you. You can develop a felt-sense of what you are offering to others, and how it may affect them. This is the basis for developing a whole-person approach. It's powerful and practical to explore your own relationship to the five layers in this book, and to take the opportunity to experience some of the practices and suggestions in each.

You'll also get a better sense of your own constitution, and see how this is like or unlike that of your clients, patients or students. You will become more sensitive and intuitive in helping others when you have experience of the medicine you are administering.

As a practitioner, your excellence in helping others is underscored by a personal felt-sense of how the practices work to change your body, mind and more. To be highly effective in helping your clients to recover from insomnia or sleep problems, read or skim this book once over, then take between five days and one full week with each action chapter, each layer of the five koshas, doing the practices yourself each day. If you want six weeks of support in doing this you also have the option of completing the online course at www.sleeprecoveryyoga.com.

Personal experience means that you know how the practices work *for* you, how they work *on* you, and the changes you experience.

You will develop a more profound relationship with each client, and knowing that each person responds to practices differently, you will have some foundation for sharing.

> The Sleep Log and the various sleep sequences from Chapter 1, marked with ☑, are available to download and print from www.jkp.com/catalogue/book/9781848193918.

Chapter One

Body Recovery

This chapter offers the basics of sleep science, the physical aspects of sleep, and daily habits that can either sabotage sleep or support sleep. I've set these out in terms that are general enough to share with clients, patients and students. There are many good books dealing with sleep hygiene, sleep-rescheduling and other facets of good sleep habits, so this forms a general overview, and focuses on aspects that relate more specifically to the yoga therapy approach.

The Forces Behind Our Sleep

First, we will look at the natural processes our bodies need to undertake in order to sleep well. We'll address some of the most common ways that we might sabotage these processes with our habits, and how adapting our habits and utilizing yoga practices can actively assist with repairing the physical mechanics of sleep. Some of the information here may seem like common sense: your client may know that caffeine, light, noise, sleep and nutrition affect sleep. Sleep and wake times and bedroom environment can all make a difference as well. Considering all the habits together and relating them to sleep patterns over time can be very powerful, though the physical changes that relate to balancing the nervous system and the experience of relaxation are, in this method, more important. Relaxed, calm sleepers are less likely to awaken to ambient noise than those in a state of constant hyper-arousal.

Establishing the best sleep hygiene and habits in the world, for a person who carries a hyper-aroused psychophysiological state, can feel as pointless as 'rearranging deckchairs on the Titanic'.

I work with my clients to identify any clear sleep saboteurs and their actual sleep patterns in our first week together, introducing a time-tested insomnia recovery tool: the sleep log (also often called a sleep diary). This is a standard tool used by clinicians. The one that I have created is heavily adapted from a model offered by the National Sleep Foundation, available through its web site. Writing down habits and patterns helps to track how various factors in life can play into their experience of sleeping well or poorly. We do the sleuth work together – identifying the link between the ways in which their habits 'break' the sleep mechanisms, and the practices that help to repair these mechanisms. The information will enable you to prioritize your guidance and therapeutic approaches. When you identify the biggest potential sleep saboteurs first, you can begin some manageable behaviour change.

At a deeper physiological level, in general, three factors affect sleep: the homeostatic body-balancing sleep drive, circadian (daily cycles) rhythms and the level of activation (stress versus relaxation). We'll look at how to support sleep recovery in each area. Because we focus on physical aspects of sleep recovery in this chapter, we'll deal with the homeostatic and circadian drives here and cover practices that can establish the physical states needed to support good sleep patterns. The chapter on energy or 'prana' will go into far greater detail on nervous system activation and relaxation and how we can use breath practices, acupressure and other techniques for immediate and longer-term sleep recovery.

The Sleep Drive: Homeostasis in Action

The 'sleep drive' or homeostatic drive towards sleep refers to the tendency for our bodies to regulate themselves and maintain an internal balance. After a day of activity, we will tend to feel tired. When we have done enough activity, this drive ideally overtakes us, and when the day–night cues say it's time to sleep, we are able to fall asleep and stay asleep. However, if there is too much arousal in the nervous system, the following will occur:

- Some people may feel tired, but not feel *sleepy*, due to too much activation (tension, stress hormone) present in the body. This state has often been referred to as 'tired but wired'. While our bodies need the capacity to enter states of excitation and relaxation to maintain healthy energy levels, if a person remains in a heightened state of agitation, stress or arousal, this can inhibit their ability to shift into parasympathetic or 'rest' mode. Some people, even when given ample down-time, may find rest or relaxation difficult, with a pervasive sense of anxiety, strain, tension or fidgetiness. We deal with repairing and rebalancing our bodies' activation–relaxation system in Chapter 2.

- Some people fall asleep easily but have difficulty maintaining sleep once the body's immediately pressing physical rest needs are decreased through the first one of two sleep cycles, which we discuss below. Many people wake up in the middle of the night one or more times. This often happens when the 'drive' to sleep caused by exhaustion wears off. Remember that the deep rest that refreshes the body comes in the first cycles of sleep. We then are physically less exhausted, and if the nervous system is jangly or activated, we are more susceptible to being awakened by external stimulus, mental activity or physical tension. In later years, hormonal fluctuations due to menopause occur for women, disrupting sleep.

Instead of creating more stress around waking in the night, this programme suggests using any waking time to invest in relaxing practices and quiet contemplation. If you practise the physical yoga postures and breath work, they will build your physical capacity to maintain deeper states of sleep and rest, and resist waking when there are noises or other external stimuli.

Although some individuals experience heightened states of arousal on an episodic or sporadic basis, some who suffer sleep difficulties exist in a state of perpetual high-alert due to trauma. It may be difficult to believe that an event long past could affect their sleep in the long term but the patterning in the nervous system may say otherwise. Insomnia is one of the core symptoms of post-traumatic stress disorder (PTSD) which may develop due to catastrophic or overwhelming events, or due to complex trauma (causing complex PTSD or CPTSD), which refers to longer-term exposure to relational abuse or neglect earlier in life. It is vital to note that these influence the brain, nervous system and psychological states in ways that may actually prevent deep levels of rest as found in REM sleep. There is a special section of this book dedicated to yoga therapy for post-traumatic insomnia (see Chapter 4).

Circadian Rhythms: The Master Code

Circadian rhythms are physical, mental and behavioural changes that follow a 24-hour cycle responding primarily to light and darkness. These natural rhythms are often disrupted by the habits of modern life, which can mean that we are expecting our bodies to be alert when they have been evolutionarily programmed to be asleep, or to sleep when we command them to, regardless of the natural rhythms established over millions of years of human history.

One of the goals of a yoga therapy approach is to make *realigning with nature* feel less like punishment and more like a positive step towards living a better, more enjoyable life. Whether quickly or slowly, changing habits from those that make us 'swim upstream' in terms of getting a good night's sleep to 'going with the flow' of nature is effort well spent.

The same effort it takes to go to a cafe for a takeaway coffee can be repurposed for a sustainable recharge like a restorative pose or simple bit of meditative shut-eye. Hours in front of the TV or binge-watching a web-series 'unwinding' before bed can be transformed into 15–20 minutes of deeply effective, excellent-feeling physical unwinding with a few simple yoga poses that create the physical sensation of calm and peace.

The habits in this chapter and the practices in the next one are cued up to the circadian rhythms.

KEY POINTS

- Daytime sunlight and evening darkness trigger different reactions in the brain that signal the release of sleep and wakefulness-related hormones (neurotransmitters).

- Changes in body temperature and digestion also affect (increase or decrease) the hormones that regulate sleep.

- Aligning with the light–dark responses, and linking behaviour to what's appropriate for the time of day, helps to repair sleep.

- The yoga therapy practices in this book realign you to these daily rhythms so that it's easier to sleep at night and feel alert all day.

The Master Clock in Your Brain

Around 20,000 nerve cells in our brains band together to form a biological 'master clock' which controls our body's response to day and night/light and dark cues in our environment. Called the suprachiasmatic nucleus, or SCN, this master clock resides in the hypothalamus, just above the juncture of the optic nerves, which bring information from the eyes into the brain. In a normally functioning person, at the end of the day the fading of daylight and the rise of ambient darkness sparks a sleep-inducing chain reaction. First, the eyes take in the change from light to dark. The change is registered in the SCN, which sends a message to the pineal gland which, in turn, triggers the brain to convert a well-known brain chemical called serotonin (referred to colloquially as the happy hormone) into melatonin, the hormone that primes the brain for sleep. Melatonin acts as a sleep-inducer, making us drowsy and setting in motion a number of physiological changes that prepare the body and brain for sleep, including a decrease in core body temperature.

Light and Devices

When we don't get enough sunshine in the daytime (due to sleeping at that time or low light conditions), this throws off the natural mechanisms in the brain that use light and dark to determine waking and sleeping hours. Bright daylight is a part of the blue part of the light spectrum, which specifically triggers the 'daytime' brain response. This may also work against our sleep, when electronic screens and LED and fluorescent lights all emit light on the blue part of the spectrum that mimics daylight. We find the blue-spectrum in LED lights, televisions, computers and smartphones. This means that we may be exposing our eyes and brains to blue light late into the night, often with these bright light sources mere inches from our eyes. The red light of candlelight or soft incandescent bulbs doesn't have the same daylight effect, and increasingly, we are seeing night-time modes on new electronics to minimize blue-light emissions.

One theory is that blue-light exposure late at night can adversely affect sleep quality by tricking the brain into responding with anti-sleep cues such as inhibiting melatonin: in a way bright light is perceived by the brain as 'daytime' and can inhibit sleep. While there is evidence to suggest that blue light from electronic devices impairs sleep (Chang *et al.*, 2014), other research seems to indicate that the jury is still out. Some of the 'electronic device effect' may be down to arousal of our nervous systems and heightened brain activity involved in working or connecting socially right up until sleep time. Either way, it is wise for those who have sensitive sleep to avoid bright light and using devices in the time before sleep, allowing an hour or more between exposure and sleep.

Unplug: Managing Light and Digital Devices

- Begin turning down lights in the home an hour before bedtime if possible.

- Keep light-emitting devices as far from your eyes as possible.

- Turn down screen brightness to the lowest setting in the evening and at night. Many new devices have dimmer or 'warm light' options.

- Avoid screen time an hour or more before bed to allow the serotonin-to-melatonin conversion.

- Use a clock rather than a smartphone for a wake-up alarm.

- Read printed materials, rather than screens, using warm light at night.

- Keep social media, work and other practices that distract from sleep time out of the bedroom, concluding all activity an hour or more before bed.

Sleep disruption can occur because of changing sleep patterns, as in 'shift work'. Alternating patterns can prove very disruptive to sleep, with daytime and some dark hour work shifts, such as those of trainee doctors and flight crew. Others with purely night-work schedules may have major disruptions as well. While some people can adapt to changing patterns more easily, for those with sensitive sleep, this can be one of the biggest sleep saboteurs. If we think about it in these terms it makes perfect sense: working against millions of years of human evolution to try to reorganize the sleep–wake patterns can be a losing proposition.

Difficulties such as jetlag and seasonal affective disorder also arise when we don't have sufficient exposure to strong ambient blue-spectrum light during the day and the contrasting ambient darkness cues at night. Our bodies don't set the sleep and wake cues properly. When these light changes happen naturally with the seasons, we adapt to light and darkness changes gradually. When we travel across time zones, however, upon landing, our bodies are on a 24-hour clock set to another set of light and dark patterns, while the cues coming from our new location may be very different. The sleep mechanisms in the brain need to catch up to the environment.

For this reason, a dark bedroom is essential for sensitive sleepers. This is also the reason that many people wake before their alarm goes off – at 5am. The changes in the environment at the break of dawn can affect circadian-rhythm sensitive sleepers more strongly than others. This is not a problem if the person has gone to sleep shortly after dark, or with enough hours for sleep, but our modern world shifts wakefulness into the dark hours of the night with perilous effects.

Age and Stage of Life Affects Sleep

We sleep according to different patterns based on our life stage. First, babies enter REM sleep before non-REM sleep, have much shorter sleep cycles than adults and, because of their small tummies, new digestive apparatus and large demand for food to fuel their growth, they wake to feed very frequently. Their sleep cycles are well out of synch with adult demands. During the course of our lifetimes, post-adolescent and pre-geriatric adulthood sees a levelling out of sleep into an average pattern. However, teens are not just trying to be difficult by going to sleep late and sleeping the day away. Sleep-phase shift occurs towards the late side in many adolescents, just as sleep-phase shift is more likely to occur towards the early side in the elder population. The peak in temperature and hormonal shifts accompanying pre-menstrual days, and the hormonal fluctuations surrounding menopause, can be highly disruptive to women's sleep patterns.

Temperature

As part of the circadian rhythms of the body, body temperature changes within a normal range throughout the day (Murphy and Campbell, 1997). If all is functioning as normal, we should experience a dip in core body temperature in the time around 9–10pm, after dark and before bedtime. When we take strenuous exercise or overly hot baths or showers during this time, the rise in temperature may adversely affect sleep with temperature cues tricking the body into wakefulness. There are differing theories about whether a hot bath is sleep-promoting or sleep-inhibiting. It's best for clients to try these things for themselves, noting the effects in their sleep log. For most people, it's good sense to sleep in a bedroom that is as cool as possible without becoming cold, supporting the temperature cues towards sleep.

MOOD, SLEEP AND SELF-MEDICATING

As described earlier, our brains need to convert serotonin into melatonin to make us feel sleepy. Medical science has associated low serotonin levels in the brain with depression or low mood – which is the basis for serotonin-affecting anti-depressant drugs. Because melatonin relies on serotonin, low serotonin levels may also correspond with sleep difficulties. Some research has indicated a correlation between lower levels of serotonin and higher levels of a stress hormone called cortisol. While we need cortisol during the day to help us to stay awake and alert, when levels are too high we also experience anxiety. If there is too much cortisol in the brain at night, we have trouble getting to sleep or staying asleep. An interesting recent study has shown that levels of cortisol, as measured in saliva, decreased significantly after those in the study participated in yoga practices.

SUBSTANCE MISUSE

Those with sleep problems may use chemical or natural substances that have stimulant or depressive effects to manage the effects of inadequate sleep during the day or to promote relaxation at night. However, sleeping pills are well known to become ineffective within weeks or months. Long-term use of these and other substances may run the risk of impairing the natural sleep–wake mechanisms. Everything from coffee to cocaine, alcohol and amphetamines can be used to manage energy and mood – often to avoid uncomfortable or unmanageable sensations and feelings ranging from tiredness to grief.

SILVIA

Silvia is in her mid-fifties and since going through menopause has had difficulty sleeping. She has been on sleeping tablets for years and, as a GP, she is well aware of their diminishing effect. She can feel the benefits are now nearly non-existent, but has felt unwilling to give them up because of the reassurance that they provide. We incorporated yoga postures into her evening routine, and Silvia has been able to wean herself off the tablets slowly, replacing the placebo effect of the pills with the genuine physical sense of calm that enables her to drift into sleep more easily. Middle-of-the-night wake-ups have lessened dramatically, and when she does wake, she is able to use stretches and breath practices to get back to sleep most nights.

CAFFEINE

The most widespread sleep saboteur is caffeine. It's ironic: when sleep is elusive, and we're tired or drowsy the next day, caffeine is seen as the solution. However, for some it may actually undermine sleep at bedtime. While some people are able to drink a cup of coffee and sleep soundly directly afterwards, most people who have delicate sleep are affected by this stimulant for hours, with heightened 'activation' of the nervous system. Some people have a baseline of higher sympathetic nervous system arousal than others (detailed in Chapter 2) or may have a chemical sensitivity to caffeine. Either way, it is important to know and share with clients the basic information that caffeine has an average half-life of two and a half to six hours (Arnaud, 1987). I use four hours as a general guide. In this case, with variances for individual metabolism, about half of the dose is metabolized in four to six hours.

Look at it this way: if you drink a double espresso at 8am it's only half gone at noon, and a quarter of it is still left at 4pm. One eighth of that is still there at 8pm. By midnight it has reached negligible levels. However, if you have that same double espresso at 4pm, a single espresso is still buzzing around at 8pm, and half an espresso is still in your system at midnight. Knowledge is power – and our clients must understand the trade-offs involved in using caffeine. The mid-afternoon rest offered in the section on restorative yoga poses works wonders for those who normally drink caffeine at that time. For those clients who have given up caffeine entirely, after an initial withdrawal period involving irritability and headaches, there is most often a marked decrease in nervous system arousal, and greater ease with staying asleep – especially when combined with the practices in this book.

THOM

Thom works in a cafe in my neighbourhood. When he heard I was working on a book about sleep, he volunteered his own story and pulled out of his satchel the bottle of melatonin he takes to try to get some sleep at night.

'How well is it working?' I asked.

'Not that well' was his reply.

Knowing that he works in a cafe, my next question was: 'How many cups of coffee do you have during the day?'

'Six,' he replied. 'Maybe seven or eight.'

I asked about timings. He'd take his last cup when the cafe closed at 6pm. When I explained about the caffeine half-life, it became clear to Thom that a double espresso at cafe closing time would still activate his nervous system at midnight, in addition to the cumulative effect of the stimulant on his nervous system. He said he'd try for a week to cut way back on his coffee, and keep it to before noon. When I showed up for lunch the following week, Thom reported a dramatic improvement in his ability to get to sleep. I also explained to him that melatonin was primarily useful for jetlag sleep problems, or for use with teens or elders due to sleep-phase problems, and Thom declared that this would save him some money, enabling him to try his first yoga class.

SUGAR

Another widespread pick-me-up is refined sugar. While not as direct in its effect as caffeine, and not technically a stimulant, over-use of sugar can create a boom-and-bust energy cycle that masks a natural dip in energy levels and the genuine need for rest during the day. Using sugar for a boost instead of taking a simple rest means that the exhaustion is not addressed. In addition, over-use of refined sugar may lead to metabolic problems. There is evidence to suggest that some people wake in the middle of the night due to the hypoglaecemic effects of the sugar boom-and-bust cycle (St-Onge, Mikic and Pietrolungo, 2016).

ALCOHOL

While alcohol is initially a relaxant, there are two important ways in which it may alter our mood and brain chemistry, which can sabotage sleep. First, alcohol stimulates the release of GABA, a neurotransmitter that lowers anxiety by inhibiting fast brain waves called 'excitatory impulses'. This accounts for the initially relaxing effect of alcohol. After a short period of GABA flooding the brain, however, the brain stops producing it, leaving a gap. After the initial relaxation, the dip in GABA means that those particularly sensitive to anxiety experience feelings of anxiety or physical symptoms like heart racing or an increase in muscle tension. Without the GABA to hold down the 'excitation' impulses, they come up stronger. This is one mechanism put forward to explain the middle-of-the-night wake-ups accompanied by anxiety that many late-night drinkers have experienced. In addition, when alcohol, which is mostly sugar, is broken down by the liver, it can cause the body temperature to rise, also disturbing sleep. Cutting out or limiting alcohol strictly, and taking out pre-sleep drinking, can go a long way to rebuilding sleep maintenance. It's also essential to assess the use of any recreational drugs, as these may seem to alleviate sleep difficulties but actually break the sleep mechanisms long term. Hauri and Linde's book *No More Sleepless Nights* (1996) and other medically based books about insomnia give a fuller account of the impact of these substances on sleep.

SIMON

Simon declared that giving up wine with his wife and their friends at dinner would make life lacklustre, and he would never give it up. Given that he was sleeping decently only one night per week, he did realize however that changes were needed. Using the sleep log, Simon was able to track that, on nights when he had more than one glass of wine, he would routinely wake for at least one major episode, accompanied by a racing heart, anxious thoughts and body tension. Simon occasionally will still enjoy a glass of wine with dinner but knows that if he indulges in more than a glass, and if it's after nine, he is very likely to awaken in the night. He will benefit from a quiet walk around his house, followed by calming yoga and breathing practices that settle the tension in his body and re-establish the breathing patterns that create relaxation. He has also begun investigating, with his naturopath, the possibility of using GABA supplements to smooth out middle-of-the-night wake-ups.

Inside Sleep: We Haven't Really Switched Off

In addition to the circadian cycles, there are cycles within our sleep as well. While we're asleep, our body and brain go through a full sleep cycle in about 60 to 90 minutes. At the beginning of each cycle, we have a twilight, almost-awake stage much like when we have just fallen asleep. We dip into deeper sleep, and at the end of each cycle we come back up near the surface to begin another cycle. Inability to manage the 'almost-awake' part without actually waking up can amount to several awakenings per night. Often, a slight noise or light can rouse us from sleep. Getting to sleep and staying asleep are easier when we incorporate specific practices that re-educate the body and brain, repatterning our ability to enter and maintain the twilight, relaxation and deep-rest states.

Physical yoga postures decrease the basic level of 'arousal' so that the sleep drive is greater than the activation drive, enabling us to maintain sleep more easily. The meditation techniques outlined in Chapter 3 are among the most effective methods I've found for training the unconscious sleeping mind to tolerate environmental disruptions and fluctuations – while remaining calmly at rest.

Waves of Sleep: The Hypnogram

Those who don't get to sleep easily or wake up in the middle of the night often say things like 'I can't switch off' or 'I can't turn my mind off'. When we go to sleep, we don't switch from 'on' to 'off' like a machine does. A great deal happens when our eyes are closed. Without a power supply, a computer can't reorganize its memory, scan for viruses, or clean up the 'desktop'. However, our human bodies and brains undergo essential maintenance, repair and enhancement when we are 'powered down'.

The 'hypnogram' (sleep diagram) shows different brain wave patterns that correspond to neurological and physiological repair and reorganization during sleep. An *average* hypnogram is shown in the figure on the next page, Optimal Nightly Sleep Cycles. Each section of the U-shaped sleep cycle, called a 'stage', accomplishes slightly different things in your body and brain during the course of the night. Some body and brain activities are front-loaded into the earlier sleep cycles during the night, while other sleep stages are dominant later on. It's helpful to understand this overall pattern of sleep cycles, as different sleep problems can correspond to difficulties at the different stages.

First, whilst the *body* is mostly relaxed during sleep, the *brain* is active in several ways. There are two general categories of sleep. A state of deep 'body rest' is called non-REM sleep. In REM sleep, our eyes move quickly beneath our eyelids, as the brain is very active in 'processing' – reorganizing memory and other functions. In an adult, the sleep cycle begins with four stages of non-REM sleep, with each stage addressing different functions in the body and brain. After these four non-REM stages, every sleep cycle finishes with a period of REM sleep. Depending upon how long you're asleep, you can have up to six cycles of sleep, moving through each of the stages. Interestingly, however, depending upon how long you've been asleep, the stages in each cycle can be longer or shorter.

We can think of it this way, roughly: for adults, at the beginning of the night the sleep cycles front-load body restoration, and relatively less time is spent in REM sleep. This puts priority on body-function so that you can still exist, even on a couple of sleep cycles. This is evolutionarily beneficial because if a human was awakened by dangerous predators or unsafe conditions, the body could respond by springing into action.

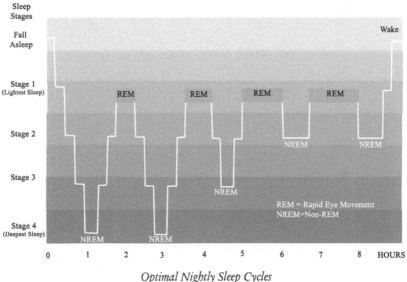

Optimal Nightly Sleep Cycles

Once the body is restored, the latter sleep stages place more emphasis on the brain-repair and restoration that's found in REM sleep. We tend to dream more and remember our dreams in the latter sleep cycles, towards the morning hours, probably due to increased time in REM sleep. When a person takes sleeping pills, this latter stage of brain wave activity, REM sleep, can be inhibited, leading to groggy/foggy mental states the following day.

The next section takes you through a full cycle of all the sleep stages.

Brain Waves and Sleep

When we're awake and active, the brain makes very small, fast, random waves called BETA waves – the nerve cells in your brain are firing in a less integrated fashion. When you relax and close your eyes, more of the nerve cells start working together, creating a more synchronous form – ALPHA waves (8–12 cycles per second). When we are sleeping, the waves get slower and 'bigger'.

- **Stage 1 sleep** exhibits a gradual transition between relaxation and sleep. Your thoughts are drifting but you are not asleep. The brain goes into a THETA wave pattern. The timing of this stage is about five to ten minutes for the average sleeper, but can be longer.

- **Stage 2 sleep** is when the brain begins to produce bursts of rapid, rhythmic brain wave activity known as sleep spindles (or K complexes). Your body temperature starts to decrease and heart rate begins to slow.

- **Stage 3 sleep** is characterized by the start of deep, slow brain waves known as DELTA waves. This transitions the brain between light sleep and a very deep sleep.

- **Stage 4 sleep** is the body of DELTA wave sleep – a deep sleep lasting about 30 minutes. This is said to be the most classically restful sleep and is concerned most with mental recovery. People deprived of this DELTA sleep or interrupted during this phase often awaken with a feeling of grogginess and that something is physically not quite right.

- **Stage 5 sleep**, also called REM sleep, is when most dreaming occurs. REM sleep is characterized by eye movement, increased breath rate and heightened brain activity. REM sleep is also referred to as paradoxical sleep because while the brain and other body systems become more active, muscles become more relaxed. While DELTA sleep seems more concerned with physical recovery, REM sleep is said to pertain more to mental recovery and processing. It's this phase of sleep that helps 'make sense of our lives'.

The in-sleep eye movement occurs as we 'look around' in our dreams. Before REM sleep, a nucleus of nerve cells in the brain stem relaxes the body's muscles in a state almost like paralysis, so that we don't move our bodies physically when we feel we are moving them in our dreams. Some people may move slightly during REM sleep, while for others the inhibition mechanism is not functioning properly and there is a lot of movement during dreams. This is considered a REM behaviour disorder, a form of parasomnia.

REM sleep normally occurs every 90 minutes on average, throughout the sleep period. The period from Stage 2 sleep to Stage 5 REM sleep is normally called one sleep cycle. As sleep continues throughout the night, each period of REM sleep lengthens. The first REM period is about five minutes, the second is about ten minutes, and the third is about 15 minutes. The final episode of REM sleep may last from 30 to 60 minutes if a person has been asleep for three or four of the 90-minute cycles. An average long-sleep is about five to six cycles per night through Stages 2 to 5.

These sleep stages relate to different brain states. One feature of sleep recovery that a holistic yoga therapy approach offers is the re-training of body and brain, which I posit gives us easier access to these states in waking and sleep. In the chapters that follow, we will recall these states and relate them to the practices that support them, including meditation and restorative poses, citing the academic/medical research evidence where possible.

The Sleep Log

In order to help recover sleep, we will need to trouble-shoot daily habits as well as repair the sleep mechanisms through yoga-based practices. We will start with information about what's happening in the client's life, using the sleep log. This tool helps clients to be more realistic about sleep and wake times, the amount of sleep they're getting and daily habits that affect sleep. It is very powerful to see daily habits laid out in one place. The Sleep Log below is available to download and print from www.jkp.com/catalogue/book/9781848193918.

☑ Table 2.1: The Sleep Log

	Monday	Tuesday	Wednesday
Sleep facts			
Wake time			
Bed time			
Sleep time (estimated time asleep)			
Wakings in night			
Total hours asleep			
Habits and experience			
Dose and timing Caffeine Alcohol Nicotine			
Amount, type and timing Exercise Rest			
Sleep recovery practices Morning Afternoon Pre-bedtime			
Daytime sleepiness			
Mood			

Thursday	Friday	Saturday	Sunday

Body Reconnection: Releasing Tension, Cultivating Interoception

The next step in sleep recovery is to reduce the pervasive effects of stress, tension, over-load and over-work. Many people who have sleep difficulties also have trouble attending to interoceptive cues – the cues that signal bodily sensations and needs. Modern occupations and lifestyles can require us to work very hard, developing habits of over-riding hunger or tiredness to keep pushing through to meet a deadline or fulfil an obligation. Over-stimulation due to information-overload seems to compound the problem, so the two are inter-related. General insensitivity to our physical bodies means that many of us ignore the signs of tiredness and push onward to when we *think* we should go to sleep – missing the important circadian rhythms' 'sleep bus'.

The Sleep Bus versus the Sleep Taxi

For people with sleep difficulties, feeling sleepy can arrive more like a bus or train than a taxi – in that sleepiness is often experienced in waves or according to a schedule, rather than accessible at any time. For many of us, if we push past the initial onset of sleepiness, we get a second wind that may carry on far longer than we wish. We may find ourselves pushing past the wave of sleepiness and then feeling wakeful much later than is conducive to a good night's sleep. Part of yoga therapy for insomnia's method of sleep recovery is training ourselves to listen to the sleepiness cues, and to get to bed when we are actually sleepy, rather than when we *think* we should go to bed. Many people keep themselves awake a lot later at night than is conducive to good sleep, by working, eating or socializing. Listening to the natural body clock can help to reset healthy sleep–wake patterns that are aligned to the circadian rhythms.

Sometimes the over-riding of one's sleepiness is not solely about daily habits. A person who has experienced abuse, neglect or trauma in early years may never have learnt how to interpret their internal body-needs cues, may have had the need to over-ride them due to neglect, or may have been forced to obey someone else's idea of what they should do rather than their own innate needs. By restoring sensitivity to the body, we help clients to effectively interpret and respond to *tiredness* and *sleepiness* cues. We can provide ways to follow these physical cues appropriately at different times of day to overcome or prevent insomnia. *Developing interoception* (internal sense of self) and *taking effective action* are concepts put forward by David Emerson (2015) in his approach to trauma-sensitive yoga. This is explored further in Chapter 4, which focuses more closely on trauma-based insomnia.

The Body Influences the Brain

From a yoga therapy perspective, we work with the communication between the body and brain as a key pathway for fostering the relaxation – and indeed the neurochemistry – needed for sleep. Through the system of afferent and efferent nerves that send messages between the musculature/viscera and the brain, bodily tension signals an 'on alert' message to the brain. In turn the brain makes the hormones that support alertness or – at its extreme – fight or flight. For example, consider the hunched-forward position created by sitting at a computer, or driving a car. When our shoulders pull forward, the ribcage contracts, resulting in something that resembles a boxer's defensive position. Breathing becomes short and uneven. The muscular tension and shorter breath are the opposite of a relaxed, open position, and you feel a difference in relaxation immediately when you take each position. The whole system responds to the tension in the body by tightening and feeling more stressed. We can dismantle the stressed-body position and signal 'calm' by gently opening the chest, stretching the intercostal muscles between the ribs, and activating the slow-acting stretch receptors in the lungs that trigger a relaxed and open state, in which we feel safe and expansive. Throughout the day we build up tension that can signal stress and prevent a sense of relaxation. The sleep sequences in this programme are specifically designed to target these 'tension hotspots' and to create a relaxed, expansive and soft body that is prepared for rest and sleep.

We know that the human body is designed to tense up, like armour, to protect us if it feels under threat. This happens before we can even think, and creates protective tension and the brain chemistry to respond to threat effectively. Physical tension can stay long after the stressful event unless it is released. Those suffering from sleep problems are often living in a physical state ranging from chronic low-level tension to chronic hyper-arousal, and the corresponding physical tension. Others may have reached complete burnout and are not in a hyper-aroused state but are hypo-aroused and can't mobilize enough energy to build up the tiredness needed to sleep.

In addition, pain can play a role in sleeplessness, and yoga can assist with alleviating pain. As we well know, pain is a warning that something's amiss. Whether it's misalignment or a stress response, persistent pain acts like the static you hear when not quite tuned in to a radio station. It is disruptive in subtle or dramatic ways, and even moderate physical discomfort can interfere with sleep. It's widely acknowledged that pain and muscular tension are hallmarks of chronic stress. While not all pain can be addressed through yoga postures, some types of muscular tension and misalignment can be addressed through yoga. For example, postures and breath work that open up tight areas like the neck, shoulders, hips and lower back can be of tremendous benefit.

The yoga sequences in this programme help to rebuild broken sleep mechanisms in different ways. Some practices are designed to pull tension out of the body to signal from body to brain 'I'm safe – I can rest', while others can get circulation going and signal wakefulness in a sustainable way. These practices build the resilience in the body that means you will not only recover your sleep, but you will cope with stress with more ease, and feel better in general. The three types of yoga asana practices (for sleep, restoration and wake-up) can be used to support the body's needs at different times of day.

These are the foundation steps upon which the other aspects of sleep recovery are built because they create palpable, self-directed change immediately, enabling a state of relaxation to occur, and empowering the client to change her state simply, without relying on other people, special props or substances.

Practices Align to Circadian Rhythms for the Desired Effect

Physical postures and stretches create different effects at bedtime, morning and afternoon as appropriate to support harmony with the day–night cycles known as circadian rhythms. Pulling tension out of the body through stretches (yoga asana) can release key muscle groups and signal relaxation in the afferent nerve messaging – from body to brain. Using postures to rest at appropriate times of day (restoratives) can help remove accumulated tiredness and decrease stress levels while leaving the drive to sleep intact so that sleep is still accessible at night. We also use physical postures to stimulate or wake up at appropriate times of day, in place of harmful, agitating, sleep-restricting or habit-forming stimulants.

Sleep recovery involves training the nervous system to relax and putting in place habits throughout the day that support you getting the rest you need, whether at night or in rest-pockets throughout the day. It is not necessary to do *all* of the practices mentioned here each day, but a well-selected combination adapted for the individual person's lifestyle can work wonders.

- Morning practice: 'mopping up' for interrupted, short or poor-quality sleep.

- Daytime (3pm slump): meditation or restorative poses in the natural 'dip' time.

- Optimal: meditation for 20 minutes am and pm – 'brain wave training' and processing the day's stressors.

- The pre-sleep buffer to wind down from the day.

- Evening practice to prepare for sleep, including the Simple or Deeper Sleep Sequence, pranayama and/or journalling.

- Managing any middle-of-the-night wake-ups with practices that discharge tension, layer in rest or build up the sleep drive to get in an additional one or two sleep cycles.

Body Recovery for Sleep: Yoga Moves

The following is an overview of the physical yoga postures which help with various aspects of sleep recovery. The most essential is the Simple Sleep Sequence. After that, for many people, the next priority is the incorporation of one restorative pose morning and/or afternoon *or* morning practices to set up the day if sleep has been elusive or insufficient. The client's needs will guide the practices you suggest, and their experience and intuition will play a role in what they keep doing.

The breath practices, meditation and mind/emotion management offered in subsequent chapters can be used in conjunction to very good effect. It is best to build in the good habits one at a time and to check that the client or student is able to find the time and space to incorporate the recommended practices.

In this chapter we explore:

- the Simple Sleep Sequence and Deeper Sleep Sequence in detail

- restorative poses in depth

- basic morning yoga poses: a suggested sequence for yoga teachers to use with clients or students

- advanced asana morning wake-up practices (for those better acquainted with a yoga practice).

The Sleep Sequences

These sequences are very carefully designed to target one or more 'tension hotspots' in the body. The general aspects included in both the Simple Sleep Sequence and the Deeper Sleep Sequence practices involve:

- breathing warm-up

- thigh stretches

- hip stretches

- hamstring stretches

- twists – supine or seated

- back-bends that support sleep

- forward folds – primarily supine.

> All of the illustrated sleep sequences that follow, marked with ☑, are available to download and print from www.jkp.com/catalogue/ book/9781848193918.

The two sequences offer variations: for those wanting a basic practice or those who may have practised yoga before, or want slightly deeper stretches.

The **Simple Sleep Sequence** is easier for people who are not already well acquainted with yoga movements. Therapists, GPs, psychiatrists and others, as well as yoga teachers, may more safely recommend these basic postures to injury-free patients: there is minimal chance of injury. You may suggest these or refer to others who may teach them. Of course, you'll need to check local insurance laws and policies first.

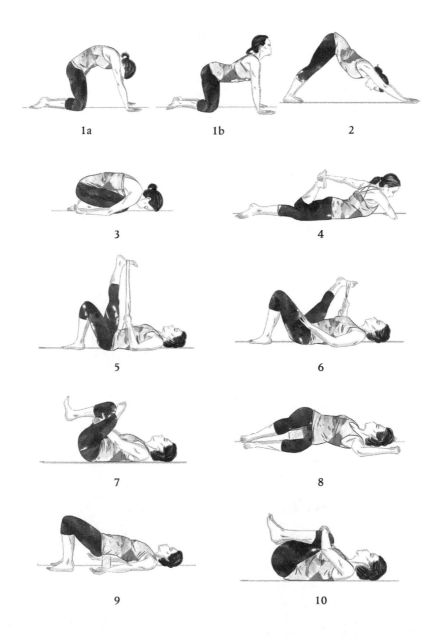

1a

1b

2

3

4

5

6

7

8

9

10

The **Deeper Sleep Sequence** is slightly more involved, in terms of postural cueing, and the poses are not as suitable for the broadest range of physical conditions. It may be more satisfying, however, to those who have been practising yoga for some time, or who have more flexible bodies. This sequence is less suitable for non-yoga teachers as the cues are more involved.

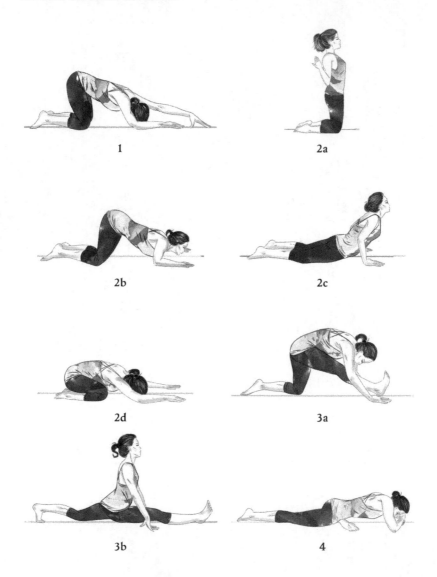

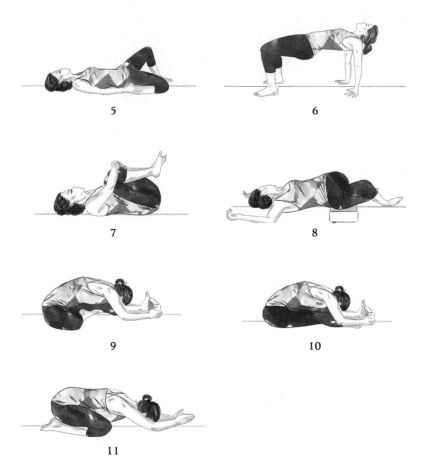

5

6

7

8

9

10

11

Daytime Yoga: Restoration and Wake Up

Restorative poses stimulate the 'relaxation response' (Benson and Klipper, 2001; Lasater, 2011). Those featured in this programme have been chosen for their effectiveness and for the relative ease of setting them up with minimal yoga props. The exception to this, requiring more in terms of props to support the body, is the 'Diamond Pose'. While this requires more setup, it is so highly effective that my students and clients love it and find it a welcome solace. These poses are used most effectively:

- in the morning to 'mop up' after a messy sleep, to start the day more rested with better physical and psychological resilience

- in the afternoon 'slump' or in the early evening, to 'put energy back on the grid' in a sustainable way, without actually sleeping, which runs the risk of diminishing the natural, much-needed evening drive towards sleep.

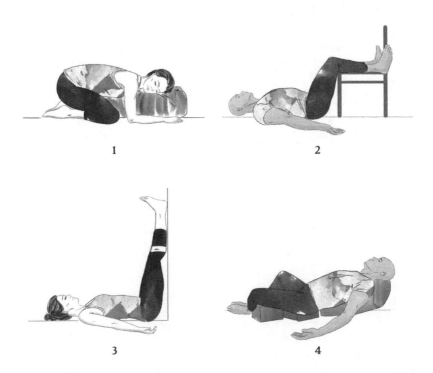

Basic morning yoga poses can empower people to boost energy sustainably. For those who have a more sedentary lifestyle or stationary workdays, morning yoga practice can be a vital resource for building the homeostatic drive towards sleep, for example expending physical energy so that it does not build up as nervous tension. These practices can also build the capacity to remain in a mildly sympathetic nervous system dominant, active state while breathing fully and evenly. Taking challenging postures, staying in alignment and taking long, even breaths builds the capacity to meet physical and mental demands with more equipoise and grace. In the next chapter, morning breath practices are provided: these complement the physical postures well, or can be used on their own if desired. The more dynamic yoga postures for **advanced asana morning wake-up** are best taught by those qualified to teach yoga or well versed in movement, physiology and other moving arts. Whereas I recommend sticking closely to the sleep sequences as they have been built very carefully, with precise attention to the purpose of each pose, the morning wake-up practices are more general guidelines for qualified teachers to use as they are or to adapt.

Morning yoga sequences can feature leg-strengthening standing postures and lunges, energizing side-body stretches, forward bends that clear the head, twists that stimulate digestion and release tension from the torso, as well as shoulder openers that lift the chest and support deeper breath. The second sequence suggestion involves deep back-bending and a version of a handstand, and so is only appropriate for those who are physically able and have practised yoga before. It is provided for those who have an established yoga practice, and as a general guide and set of ideas for those teaching active yoga.

Because offering these practices is not recommended for those who are not already qualified to teach yoga, the morning practice section offers minimal cueing/step-by-step instructions, and instead offers an overview of suggested postures.

☑ SIMPLE SLEEP SEQUENCE

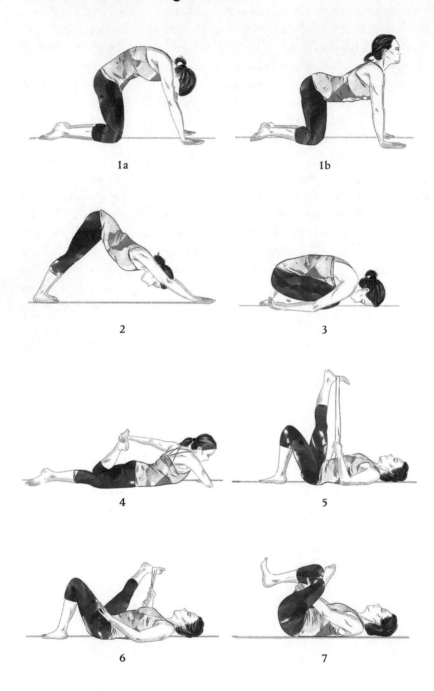

1a

1b

2

3

4

5

6

7

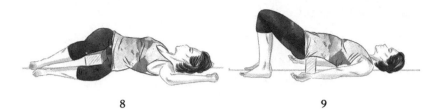

8   9

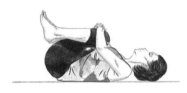

10

These poses are intended to be practised either on the floor or on the bed. The following sections describe the Simple Sleep Sequence step by step:

1. Cat/Cow Stretches

2. Downward-Facing Dog Pose (Optional)

3. Child's Pose – Calming Back Stretch

4. Simple Thigh Stretch – Half Frog Pose

5. Extended Leg Stretch – Hamstring/Back of Thigh Stretch

6. Extended Inner Thigh Stretch

7. Outer Hip Stretch – 'Threading the Needle'

8. Simple Supine Spinal Twist

9. Supported Little Bridge Pose

10. Knees to Chest Pose – Supta Balasana

1. Cat/Cow Stretches

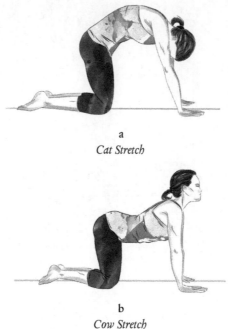

a

Cat Stretch

b

Cow Stretch

Benefit

This pose stretches the intercostal muscles and shoulders, adding space to the breathing practice. It is therefore very beneficial to begin a sleep practice with this. To keep it relaxed, make sure that the eyes are relaxed as the chin stretches upward.

Step by Step

- Come onto an all fours/hands and knees position.

- Keep both wrists under shoulders and knees under hips, keeping the hands and feet aligned and alert.

- As you inhale, lift the chest, while arching the back. This brings breath into the front of the lungs.

- As you exhale, draw the navel towards the spine, pressing the breath out.

- Repeat a few times with a relaxed expression on your face.

2. Downward-Facing Dog Pose (Optional)

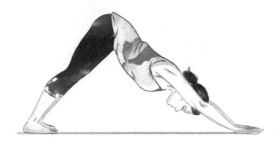

Benefit

This pose re-establishes good circulation and combats stagnant breathing. Placing your head below your heart calms the mind, and being upside down brings circulation to the arms and chest. This pose also stretches out the hamstrings and lengthens the spinal muscles.

Step by Step

- From an all-fours position, lift your knees off the floor, keeping everything else the same.

- Press your hips upwards and back, making an inverted V shape, so that your bottom is in the pinnacle of the inverted V shape.

- Keep your arms straight and fingers spread evenly, with equal weight into all parts of the hand.

- Keep your chest pressing back towards your thighs, to keep pressure off your shoulders.

3. Child's Pose – Calming Back Stretch

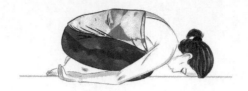

Benefit

This pose is gently restorative, calming the body and mind. It stretches out the long muscles that line your spine and provides both a gentle hip opener and stretch for the front of the legs and tops of the feet.

Step by Step

- Come onto an all fours/hands and knees position.

- Place your big toes together and knees apart.

- Bring your bottom down towards your heels. If this is too much strain on your hips, you can roll up a blanket and place it beneath your bottom.

- If your head doesn't reach the floor you can use a blanket or yoga block underneath. With your forehead in the downward position, press the flesh of your forehead downward to calm the nervous system.

- Breathe here: breathe up the back of your body and down the front of your body. Stay here for five to ten breaths, or longer if you wish.

4. Simple Thigh Stretch – Half Frog Pose

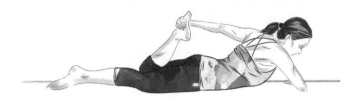

Benefit

This pose stretches the thigh (quadriceps) muscle – one of the largest muscles in the body. When this muscle is tight it can create tension in the low back, either directly or through its effect on the hamstrings, at the other side of the femur bone, or in tightening the hip flexor just above the thigh muscle. Because this pose stretches the biggest, thickest muscle in the body, bringing blood flow into the muscle, circulation there improves, creating a downward grounding effect.

Step by Step

- Lie down in a face-down position with your belly on the floor with the tops of your feet pressing into the floor.

- Bring your right forearm parallel to the front edge of your mat, lifting your shoulders and chest away from the floor.

- Bend your left knee and reach your left hand back to hold the top of the left foot.

- Keep the left side of your torso long by breathing deeply and extending your body.

- Squeeze the thighs toward the midline of your body, keeping the left knee in line with your sitting bone to keep the knee in good alignment and protect your back.

- Pull your low belly away from the floor and direct your bottom down towards the heels to remove some of the curve in the lower back. This will move the stretch deeper into the front of the thigh.

- To create a dynamic tension that stretches the muscle further, press the left foot back into your left hand as you draw that same left foot forward towards your bottom.

- Repeat on the other side.

After doing each side of the thigh stretch, flip over onto your back for the next set of postures, which will complete the sequence.

5. Extended Leg Stretch – Hamstring/ Back of Thigh Stretch

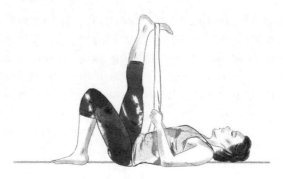

Benefit

This pose stretches and releases the hamstrings, and balances the circulation in the legs and belly. It helps to alleviate tension in the back and is grounding in its effect. Because you lift your leg up and foot up, it helps to dispel fluid retention in the legs.

Props

A yoga belt, robe/dressing gown belt or tie.

Step by Step

- Lie down on your back with your knees bent and the soles of your feet on the floor.

- Keep your lower back gently curved, so that the natural arch is present in the spine, leaving a little space between the lower back and the floor.

- Extend your right leg up towards the ceiling and push the ball of your foot into the belt, keeping the knee unlocked.

- Draw down on the belt with your hands, *keeping your elbows on the floor with your shoulders relaxed.*

- Press the thigh bone away from your chest so the leg straightens more – and keep breathing into your lower belly. Every exhalation will enable you to stretch a bit deeper.

This pose and the next two (Poses 5, 6 and 7) work together on each side. Continue the next two poses on the right side, before doing this same pose on the other side. You will do three poses in a row – 5, 6 and 7 on the right, and then do poses 5, 6 and 7 on the left side. Incorporate a pause between doing the poses on the right side and moving on to the second side. In this pause, feel the difference between your right and left sides. If you don't feel much of a difference, you may either need to:

- breathe more deeply, slowly and calmly as you stretch

- add more resistance (e.g. engage your muscles and then press outward to lengthen the muscles more).

6. Extended Inner Thigh Stretch

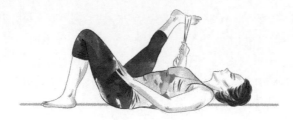

Benefit

This pose releases the inner thighs/hamstrings, opening the hip area. This can have a deeply relaxing effect by allowing the muscles around the hip and pelvis to relax. It promotes better circulation into the lower belly and pelvis.

Props

A yoga belt, robe/dressing gown belt or tie.

Step by Step

- Take both ends of the belt into your right hand with your right foot extended up into the belt.

- Place your other hand on your hip to help keep the pelvis even, so the lower back and grounded side bottom don't lift away from the floor.

- Don't try to get the extended leg all the way to the floor if this causes the pelvis to tilt, and the opposite side buttock lifts off the floor.

- Keep arms relaxed and elbows resting on the floor as you pull back on the belt with your hand.

Move on to the next pose (Pose 7) before moving on to the second side.

7. Outer Hip Stretch – 'Threading the Needle'

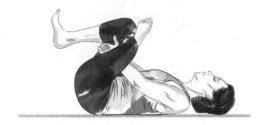

Benefit

This stretches the outer hip, which releases the lower back, opening the nerve pathways into the lower belly organs, as well as the inner thigh and sacral (lower back) area. Excellent for those who sit in chairs all day, drive or travel a lot.

Step by Step

- Lying on your back with the low back gently curved, cross your right ankle over the top of your left knee at the bottom of the thigh.

- Flex your top foot to engage the calf muscle and protect the knee.

- Wrap the top hip downward, moving the sitting bone in your bottom down towards the tailbone which is at the centre of the bottom.

- Draw in the lower knee towards your chest to intensify the stretch.

- Resist away with the rotated leg by moving your hip down, rather than pressing into your knee.

Between this hip stretch and doing Poses 5, 6 and 7 on the second side, pause to integrate the difference in sensation between the side just stretched and the one that has not yet been stretched. This interoception (body awareness) pause can be very valuable in that the student or client can come to feel the difference between even a mildly tense and a more relaxed physical state.

8. Simple Supine Spinal Twist

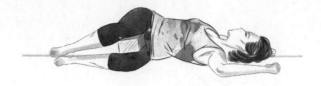

Benefit

This pose releases the muscles along the thoracic spine, in the middle back, and relaxes the upper back/shoulders. It opens the chest and expands the breathing space by stretching the diaphragm. It works particularly well with the middle-ribcage breath explained as part of three-part breathing in the next chapter. This enables the chest to expand and soften more freely. This pose also opens and relaxes the 'solar plexus' area near the stomach which often carries anxiety and tension. Finally, it also lengthens the hard-to-stretch muscles that connect the lower back to the shoulders. Twists gently compress and then release the internal organs, flushing them and removing tension in the belly.

Props

A yoga block or firm cushion.

Step by Step

- Roll completely to your right side.

- Bend knees up to the same height as the hips, placing the outer right hip bone on the floor.

- Stack the left leg evenly on top of the right, so that the knees match. Squeeze a yoga block or cushion between the knees to keep the sacro-iliac (lower back) joints even.

- Keeping the lower body stable in this position, twist from the middle/upper back, moving the right shoulder to the right.

- Press the shoulder down towards the floor, breathing into the upper back to broaden there.

- Posture tip: the block between the knees helps keep the knees in line, and keeps the lower back even. This is especially good for people with lower back concerns/pain.

Do this on the second side before moving on to Pose 9.

9. Supported Little Bridge Pose

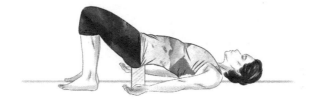

Benefit

This pose opens the breath into the chest, stretches the pectoral muscles, opens the diaphragm and lengthens the often-contracted belly muscles. This also brings circulation into the throat, where the thyroid and parathyroid reside. These two glands are associated with hormonal regulation, including digestion and sleep. This pose may work by putting pressure on the 'baroreceptors' located at the top of the lungs which intensifies the 'relaxation response'.

Props

A yoga block or thick book.

Step by Step

- Lie on your back with knees bent, soles of the feet to the floor and knees pointing up to the ceiling.

- Place your ankles directly under your knees, feet parallel.

- Posture alignment tip: if heels are too close to the buttocks the pelvis and hip flexors will contract. If feet are too far from the buttocks the pose becomes less stable.

- Keep tummy muscles gently engaged.

- Lift your hips while keeping your inner thighs and bottom evenly engaged but not gripping. Powering up your legs will support your lower back.

- Draw your shoulder blades towards the centre of your back. Keep the sides of your body long so you can breathe freely.

- Posture tip: keep the back of your neck free with its natural curve. Don't flatten the back of the neck as this can cause injury and creates tension in the face.

- Rest your low back on a yoga block on its lowest or middle 'setting', meaning that your hips are lifted two to five inches above the floor. You can use a firm cushion or books. For the relaxation effects of this pose, your hips must be substantially below the level of your knees.

10. Knees to Chest Pose – Supta Balasana

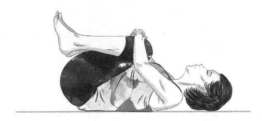

Benefit

This pose creates a gentle, even balance to the back-bending action of the Supported Little Bridge Pose and can feel soothing and containing. Child's Pose may be substituted at this point.

Step by Step

- Lying on your back, draw your knees inward towards your chest and take several breaths to lengthen the lower back.

- Option: if practising on the floor instead of a bed, some small slow circular rolls gently pressing the low back into the floor may feel relaxing.

- Place your palms on your kneecaps and let your legs drop away from your torso as much as possible without losing your grip.

- Roll in small circles to release tension in the muscle-to-bone connections along the sacrum, which supports relaxation and grounding.

☑ DEEPER SLEEP SEQUENCE

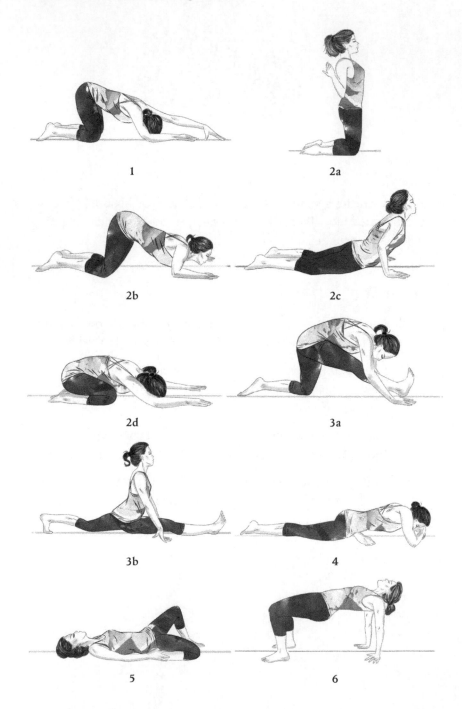

1

2a

2b

2c

2d

3a

3b

4

5

6

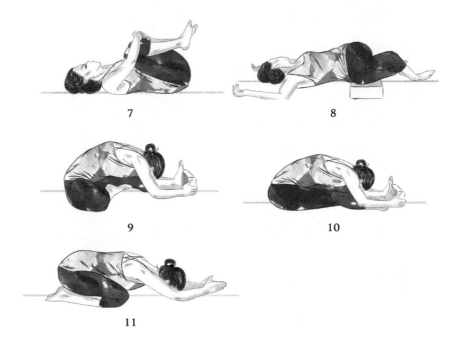

7

8

9

10

11

This is a practice for more experienced yogis or those who are more at home with the moves: it relies on a bit more flexibility in the legs and hips. As with the Simple Sleep Sequence, it should be practised in the evening to prepare for bed and can be practised on the floor or on the bed.

1. Extended Child's Pose – Side Stretch

2. Earth Salutation (Integrates Four Poses)

    a. Kneeling with Torso Upright

    b. All Fours Pose

    c. Low Cobra Pose

    d. Extended Child's Pose

3. Hamstring Stretch

    a. Runner's Lunge

    b. Hanumanasana Splits (Optional Variation)

4. Pigeon Hip Stretch

5. Half Hero Pose (Virasana)

6. Tabletop Pose

7. Knees to Chest Pose – Supta Balasana

8. Cross-Legged Supine Twist

9. One-Legged Forward Bend – Janu Sirsasana

10. Two-Legged Forward Bend – Paschimotanasana

11. Extended Child's Pose (Optional Bolster)

1. Extended Child's Pose – Side Stretch

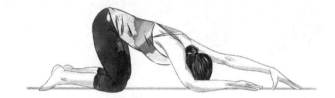

Benefit

This pose stretches the muscles between the ribs and lengthens the spinal muscles on each side, giving a feeling of space and enabling the breath to flow more freely.

Step by Step

- Come onto an all fours/hands and knees position.

- Place your right elbow on the floor, and drop your head to your right forearm.

- Reach your left hand and arm across to the right front corner of your mat, to stretch the left side of your torso.

- Keep your left hip pressing back to increase the stretch.

- Breathe into the back of the waistline and ribcage and feel the stretch along the left side of your body. Repeat on the other side.

2. Earth Salutation (Integrates Four Poses)

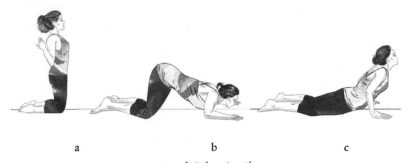

a   b   c

Earth Salutation Flow

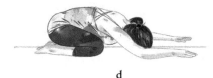

d

Earth Salutation Extended Child's Pose

a. Kneeling with Torso Upright

a. All Fours Pose

b. Low Cobra Pose

c. Extended Child's Pose

Benefit

This series of poses creates a gently dynamic flow, as it moves rhythmically with the inhalation and exhalation to initiate the movements. It engages the major muscles of the arms and legs, so that they are more integrated and more evenly activated, which helps to create the perfect conditions for deeper release. This series also opens the chest with its High Cobra Pose.

Step by Step

- Start on your knees with your torso lifted up, inhale and take your hands in prayer to your third eye point – the space between the brows.

- Exhale. Send your hands to the floor with your exhale, placing hands and knees on the floor in all-fours position/hands and knees. Take an in-breath here.

- Exhale. Place your belly and legs on the floor.

- Inhale. Lift your chest to arch forward into Cobra Pose.

  - Keep your elbows wide, so you're not lifting your arms up.

  - Slide your chest forward and through, lengthening forward rather than crunching in the lower back.

  - Stay for one to two more breaths if desired.

- Exhale and finish the Earth Salutation by moving your hips back to your heels in Child's Pose.

3. Hamstring Stretch

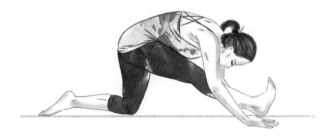

a
Runner's Lunge

Benefit

This stretches the long muscles that connect from the knee to the sitting bones in the bottom, which helps to release the lower back and create a more balanced circulation in the pelvis.

Step by Step

- From an all-fours position, step your right foot forward, straightening your right leg, with heel on the floor and toes pointed towards the ceiling.

- Keep your hands on either side of your right leg, fingertips or hands to the floor or resting on blocks or bricks.

- Repeat on the other side.

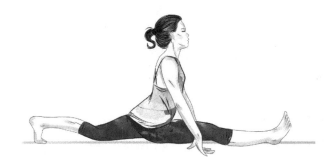

b

Hanumanasana Splits (Optional Variation)

Benefit

This pose deepens the hamstring stretch above, and involves balancing the pelvis by activating and squeezing the pelvic floor and outer hip muscles as well as the low abdominals. It is a very deep hamstring stretch that requires balance between two sides of the pelvis and can be a powerful release of tension for those who access this easily.

Step by Step

- Keep the position above with your front leg straightening and walk your back knee and foot back behind you further.

- Extend from the lunge position towards Hanumanasana/Splits Pose. This is a variation on the pose above, and you inch by inch move your back leg back; in between each movement, reintegrate your hips, belly and pelvic floor, keeping your hips pointed forward as much as possible.

4. Pigeon Hip Stretch

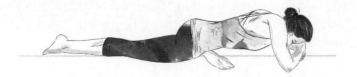

Benefit

This deep hip stretch can be very relaxing to the nervous system, and the forward-bending action turns the mind inward easily. It releases tension from the lower back by lengthening and releasing the piriformis, gluteal and adductor muscles.

Step by Step

- Start on hands and knees in all-fours position.

- Drag your right knee on the floor towards your right wrist.

- Flip your right foot in front of your left thigh.

- Extend your left leg back to lengthen it away from your torso.

- Lift up and lengthen through your chest.

- Squeeze the two sides of your hips evenly.

- Bow forward, placing your elbows and forearms to the floor, keeping the leg position, and stabilize your pelvis to the centre.

- Keep pressing back through your left leg and engaging your pelvic floor to stabilize the two sides of the hips.

- Breathe deeply in, and out, in a relaxed way, allowing your body to deepen into the stretch particularly on the exhale.

- Repeat on the other side.

5. Half Hero Pose (Virasana)

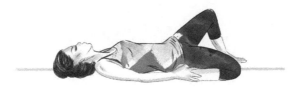

Benefit

This is a very deep thigh stretch for the 'bottom' leg which bends back at an extreme angle. If you have tender, painful or problematic knees, you may wish to do the thigh stretch from the Simple Sleep Sequence or be sure to do this pose with your bottom/buttocks resting on a high block to decrease the knee strain – and don't come all the way down to rest your shoulders on the floor.

Step by Step

- From a kneeling position sit back between your heels, using a block under your bottom if this causes any strain.
- Press the tops of your feet into the floor, toenails to floor.
- To stretch the right thigh more deeply, step your left foot out, using your left foot to brace you on the floor, by pressing the sole of your left foot to the floor with your left knee pointing towards the ceiling.
- Press your right foot down into the floor and breathe deeply, stretching from your right knee through your right thigh into your belly.
- You might drop your elbows to the floor and arch your back, lifting your chest into a gentle backbend. Do keep your hips even and support your low back by engaging the abdominal muscles.
- You can press into your left foot and lift your left side bottom off the floor to move gently side to side to stretch the right thigh muscles.
- Come back up into all-fours position.
- Repeat on the other side.

6. Tabletop Pose

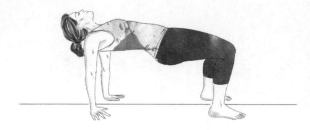

Benefit

This pose opens the breath into the chest, stretches the pectoral muscles, opens the diaphragm and lengthens the often-contracted belly muscles. This also brings circulation into the throat, where the thyroid and parathyroid reside. These two glands are associated with hormonal regulation, including digestion and sleep. Please note: if you are practising this sequence on your bed, please take care with this pose. If the bed is not firm enough, it may cause compression in your wrists. You may wish to do this pose on the floor to distribute weight evenly through your hands and wrists.

Step by Step

- Sit with your legs out in front of you and place the soles of your feet on the floor with knees bent to point upwards to the sky. Position the base of your second toe, front of ankle, knee and hip point in a straight line with both feet parallel.

- Place your hands behind, with your fingers turned outward away from your body, and lift up your chest to lengthen your back.

- While pressing your feet firmly into the floor, lift your hips, keeping your bottom engaged but not gripping. Power up your legs to support your lower back and use your pelvic floor and tummy muscles to support you. This will protect your back – it should be a bit of an effort.

- Position your body so that your torso is lifted up and parallel to the floor, and your arms and legs hold you up.

- If you have the ability to turn your fingers towards your heels, you may deepen the arm stretch in this way.

- Lengthen the sides of your torso so that you can breathe freely.

- Lean your head back so that it extends out from the rest of your spine but do not flip your head back, as doing so will make it harder to breathe and can strain your neck.

- Keep your chest open and do not sink your chest down, which will hunch your shoulders. Stay in the pose only if you can keep your chest lifted.

- Build your tolerance for this pose slowly, starting with 15 seconds and working up to one minute or more with long smooth breathing that lifts the chest.

- Lie down on your back with the soles of your feet on the floor and your knees up after practising this pose – allow the effects to be felt.

7. Knees to Chest Pose – Supta Balasana

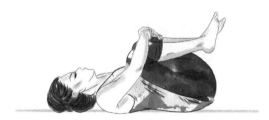

Benefit

This pose feels soothing and containing. You may choose to substitute Child's Pose at this point as it also feels very contained and calming.

Step by Step

- Lying on your back, draw your knees inward towards your chest and take several breaths to lengthen the spine.

- If practising on the floor instead of a bed, some small slow rolls on the low back can be very deeply relaxing.

8. Cross-Legged Supine Twist

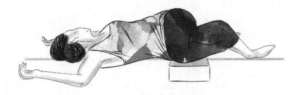

Benefit

This pose releases the muscles along the middle back, relaxing the upper back/shoulders. It opens the chest and expands your breathing space. The lungs can move more freely. It also opens the 'solar plexus' area near the stomach, which often carries anxiety and tension. This also lengthens the hard-to-stretch muscles that connect the lower back to the shoulders. Twists gently compress and then release the internal organs, with a feeling as though they are 'flushing' them and removing tension in the belly.

Props

A yoga block or cushion.

Step by Step

- Lie on your back with your knees bent and arms out wide at shoulder height.

- Hook the right leg completely over the left, twisting. The legs hug strongly together. If you have any low back pain, just stack the legs up rather than crossing them.

- Roll completely to the outer right hip with the hip bone on the floor.

- Twist from the middle/upper back, moving the right shoulder to the right and let the left shoulder drop towards the floor.

- You can put a block underneath the knee so that you're supported there and you can lengthen through the left side more fully.

- Bring your knees back into centre, uncross the legs and then come to the second side.

- After the second side, you can repeat Knees to Chest Pose before taking the next pose.

9. One-Legged Forward Bend – Janu Sirsasana

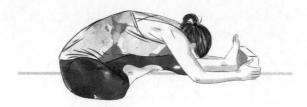

Benefit

This pose is an excellent counterpose to the leg lengtheners at the start of this series, mirroring the deep hamstring stretch. The pose is calming and cooling, and releases the major muscle chains. It also helps prepare for the following forward bend.

Step by Step

- Sit upright on the floor.

- Bring your right foot into your groin, rotating the right knee out to the side. Extend your left leg out in front. You can bring your block to the outside of the right knee side if it needs a little support if the groin is gripping or if your right knee is hovering above the floor.

- Move your torso forward over your left leg, and place your hands either side of your left leg, or move them towards your foot.

- If you have a lot of flexibility in the hamstring, you can move your hands to your left foot as you bend forward.

- Stay here for five breaths, inhaling and exhaling deeply and smoothly.

- As you inhale, come up to sit.

- Change to the second side.

10. Two-Legged Forward Bend – Paschimotanasana

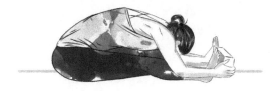

Benefit

This stretches out the spinal nerves, the spinal muscles and the hamstrings. It can also stretch into the calves very deeply. The lengthening through the back of the neck and lower back also tends to have calming effects.

Props

Yoga block.

Step by Step

- Sit with your legs extended straight forward.
- Place the block between your calves.
- Fold forward at the waist, elongating your chest forward.
- Stretch your legs out as straight as possible.
- Put your elbows on the block, and you can place your hands in prayer position, gliding the skin of the forehead downward to relax.
- Hug your belly in to support your back, lengthening. As you exhale, hug your shins.
- If you need to keep your hands on the floor and the arms straight, that's fine here.
- Take time to breathe in and out deeply and evenly.
- If you get that far down, you can rest your forehead on the block.

- Again, you can use the block at the feet if you need a much deeper stretch.

- As you inhale, come up to sit.

11. Extended Child's Pose (Optional Bolster)

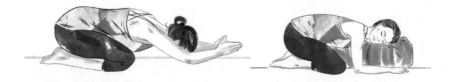

Benefit

This pose is gently restorative, calming the body and mind. It is an inward-folding finishing pose for the Deeper Sleep Sequence.

Props

Bolster or rolled-up blanket.

Step by Step

- Come onto an all fours/hands and knees position.

- Place your big toes together and knees apart, bringing the sitting bones down towards your heels.

- Place a bolster or rolled-up blanket between your legs in line with your torso and lay your torso and head onto the bolster/blanket.

- Breathe here: breathe up the back of your body and down the front of your body. Stay here for five to ten breaths, or longer if you wish.

This completes the Deeper Sleep Sequence.

☑ RESTORATIVE POSES

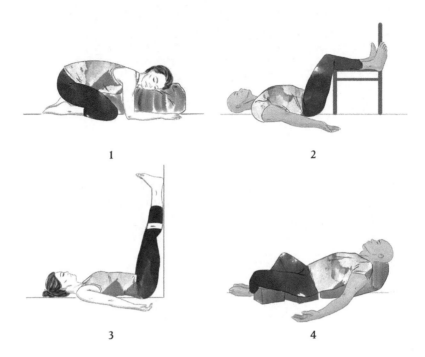

These poses have been modified and simplified from the style of restorative yoga taught by Judith Lasater (2011), which I used in my personal practice and have adapted for use with my insomnia clients and students, minimizing the use of props and setup to make them as easily accessible and practical as possible.

1. Child's Pose

2. Legs-Up Pose Using a Chair or Wall

3. Legs Up the Wall (Optional Variation)

4. Restorative Goddess Pose/Diamond Pose/Deluxe Pose

1. Child's Pose

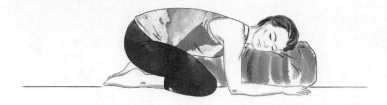

Benefit

This pose stretches out the front of the legs and lower back. It brings your attention inward, resting the eyes, face and shoulders. The posture gently brings better circulation into the belly and lungs as the blood flows downward with gravity. It can feel like a tremendous relief after a depleting day to come 'home'.

Props

A bolster, cushion or rolled-up blanket.

Step by Step

- Come onto an all fours/hands and knees position.

- Place your big toes together and knees apart, bringing the sitting bones down towards your heels. If this is too difficult you can roll up a blanket and place it beneath your bottom.

- Place your torso and head on a bolster or rolled-up blanket.

- Breathe here: breathe up the back of your body and down the front of your body. Stay here for five to ten breaths, or longer if you wish.

2. Legs-Up Pose Using a Chair or Wall

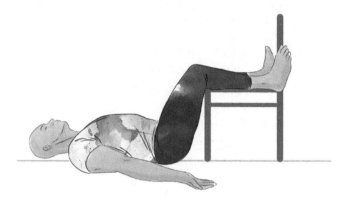

Benefit

For many people, this pose quiets the mind and generally relaxes the body. The version with calves on the seat of a chair is one of my favourites for the middle of the day – and I find even just a few minutes can feel like an energy-reset. It's known to lower blood pressure and refresh tired legs. It can be done at the end of an active practice to rejuvenate, as part of a restorative series, or by itself during a busy day. Avoid this pose if you are menstruating or pregnant or if you have gastric reflux or heart disease.

Props

Use a chair with stable (non-rolling) base for the chair version, or a sofa with its seat low enough so that you can rest your shins on it comfortably.

Step by Step

- Approach a chair or sofa and lie down on your back.

- Swing the back of your calves onto the sofa cushions or seat of the chair.

- Place a rolled-up towel or blanket under the curve of your neck or a low cushion to support your head if needed.

- If your shins roll out, this can create tension in your lower back, so you can tuck your shins into a blanket or use a belt to hold them at hip distance apart.

- Posture tip: move your bottom away from the seat of the chair or sofa so that you maintain a gentle curve in your lower back. Make sure that the hip flexor crease – where your legs meet your torso – is hollow. When you are in the optimal position, your legs will relax, with the head of the thighbone nestling into the back of the pelvis, and this will relax the lower back. Adjust until this feels comfortable.

- Stay here with palms facing upward and arms out to the sides or resting gently on the tummy if that feels safer or more comfortable.

- Make sure that the chin is slightly lower than the forehead, without tensing the back of the neck. The best position for relaxation of the head and neck is when the back of the skull, rather than the neck, is resting on the floor.

3. Legs Up the Wall (Optional Variation)

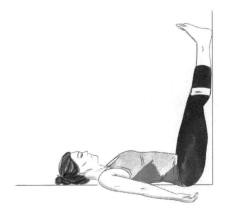

- This pose can be done with legs up the wall. It's vital to keep the bottom far away enough from the wall so that there is no tension in the hips and hamstrings, and close enough so that the legs are supported.

- For this I often place a firm cushion under the sacrum/low back, and place a belt looped firmly around the shins.

- Maintain the gentle arch in the lower back and relaxation at the hip flexor crease – if the pubic bone is higher than the front pelvic bones (called the anterior superior iliac spine or ASIS), then the pose will be less relaxing, and breathing is not as free.

- When the legs relax in this position, they often drop out to the sides, which can create tension in the lower back and groin. The belt holds everything in place and allows the hip flexors to relax, because they don't have to stabilize the legs.

4. Restorative Goddess Pose/ Diamond Pose/Deluxe Pose

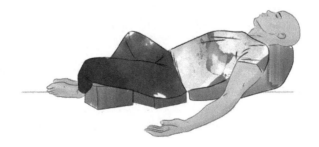

Benefit

This pose is an essential power-down: a restoring and replenishing pose. It can be used in the morning to 'mop up' after insufficient rest or in the afternoon for a deep rest to recharge without caffeine or sugar. Its standard yoga name is supta baddha konasana (Supine Bound Angle Pose) but this is often translated as 'Goddess Pose'. To make it more gender-neutral and memorable, I call it Diamond Pose or Deluxe Pose.

Props

Get a bolster, as well as something stable to prop the bolster up on an incline, and at least two blocks or blankets, which will be used for support under the thighs in order to release the grip of the hip flexors and protect the knees. Most people will also require a cushion, folded blanket or flat block under the bottom to decrease the curve in the lower back.

Step by Step

- Place a bolster or firm cushion on an incline of up to 45 degrees.

- Set up a cushion, block or folded blanket at the lower short end of the bolster.

- Sit with your bottom on this and lie the spine along the bolster's length, with the head at the top of the bolster.

- Make sure that the back of the skull is completely supported. You may need to put a folded blanket under the back of the skull. It is important that the forehead does not tilt upwards here. It should remain flat or with the forehead slightly higher than the eyes.

- Place the soles of the feet together with the knees bent outward, in an external rotation. Bring the feet as far away from the torso as possible. This decreases the strain on the knees and hip flexors and creates a more relaxed position.

- Place support under the upper thighs with blocks. These should be high enough so that there is no tightness where the torso and thighs join.

- If possible, place folded blankets or blocks under the forearms, to decrease strain on the shoulder joints.

- Stay in this position to release into deeper relaxation, for up to 20 minutes.

- If it is difficult to relax here initially, you may wish to try three-part breathing as a lead-in to releasing into the posture.

Energising Morning Yoga Poses

A morning practice of yoga postures can awaken and energize the body and enliven the mind. Getting breath and circulation on-stream can create greater clear-headedness in preparation for the day ahead. Important features of a morning practice include:

- opening the shoulders

- stretching the ribcage

- bringing the heart and lungs into an inverted (downward-facing) position

- lower body stability poses, creating a sense of focus and direction

- hip and thigh stretches, promoting grounding, meaning that the energetic quality is also steady at the same time.

This set of suggested morning poses utilizes some of the same postures indicated as helpful for sleep, but they are done early in the day, in a different order, with variations and combined with different breath practices. You will notice that instead of being close to the floor there is more up and down, and more vigorous transitions between poses, as well as standing and inversion (going upside down).

1. Cat/Cow Stretches

2. Extended Child's Pose – Side Stretch

3. Downward-Facing Dog Pose with Optional Alternating Leg Stretches

4. Forward Fold – Prasarita Padottanasana

5. Side-to-Side Forward Fold

6. Lunge Poses

7. Pyramid Pose

8. Extended Side Angle with Twist

9. One-Leg Downward-Facing Dog (to Counterpose Twists)

10. Pigeon Hip Stretch

11. Little Bridge Pose – Setubandha

12. Seated Side Twist

13. Sukhasana (Easy Pose)

☑ BASIC MORNING YOGA POSES

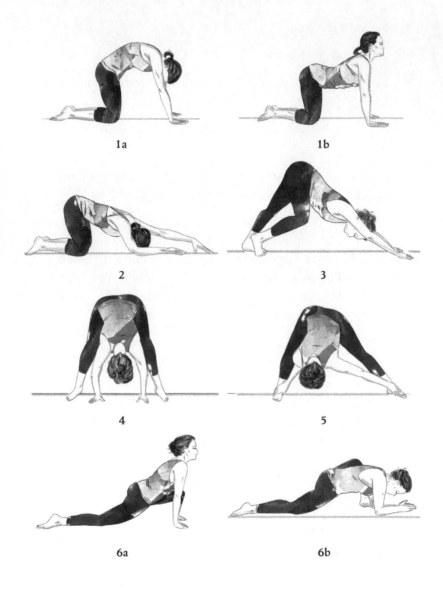

1a   1b

2   3

4   5

6a   6b

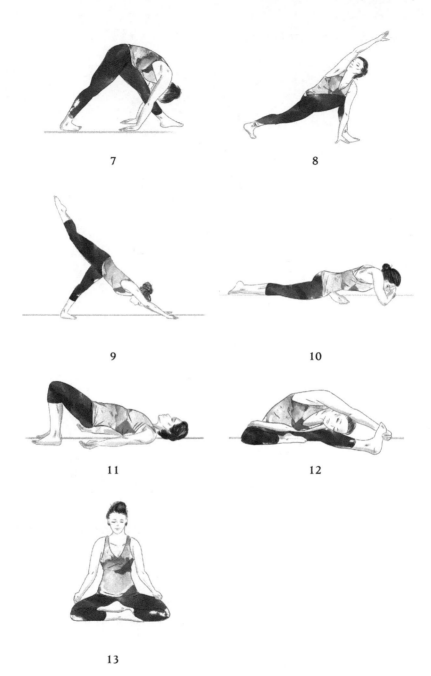

1. Cat/Cow Stretches

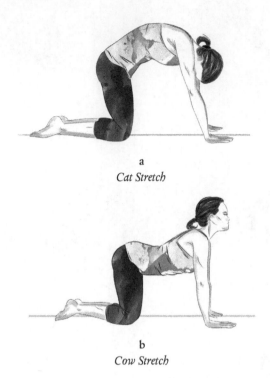

a

Cat Stretch

b

Cow Stretch

Benefit

Moving back and forth between these poses stretches the muscles along the ribcage and shoulders, adding space to your breath. They also tone and stretch one of the key nerves that promotes mental health and wellbeing – the vagus nerve – which runs from the back of the skull through the length of the torso. To keep it relaxed, make sure that the eyes are relaxed as the chin stretches upward.

2. Extended Child's Pose – Side Stretch

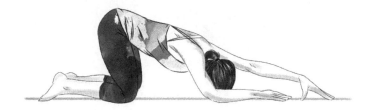

Benefit

This pose stretches the intercostal muscles on the sides of the ribs. You'll feel more spacious when you breathe more freely. The stretch receptors in the chest lengthen, signalling from the body to the brain a sense of openness, alertness and safety.

3. Downward-Facing Dog Pose with Optional Alternating Leg Stretches

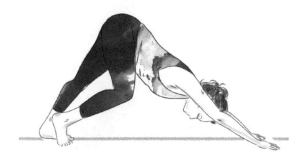

Benefit

This pose charges up the arms, which hold strong. It brings circulation into the front of the lungs and chest, which is awakening and stimulating. The moving of one heel down at a time stretches the back of the calf and back of the thigh, which have grounding and steadying effects.

4. Forward Fold – Prasarita Padottanasana

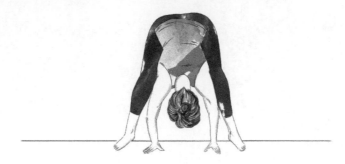

Benefit

This deep forward bend releases the shoulders and stretches the long spinal muscles, allowing more space for the spinal nerves, helping your body and brain communicate more effectively. It also provides a gentle hamstring stretch when the knees are bent and you slowly straighten your legs. The forward-bending effect continues to wake up your body gently.

5. Side-to-Side Forward Fold

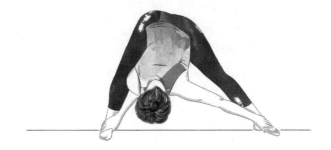

Benefit

This pose increases strength and circulation in the legs while energizing the lungs and stretching the spinal muscles and ribcage.

6. Lunge Poses

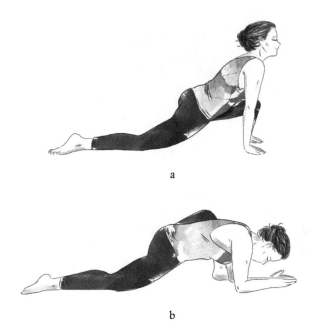

a

b

Benefit

Lunges are brilliant for stretching the back thigh, as it lengthens to the back of the mat. They also increase strength in the gluteal muscles, and cultivate abdominal strength for stability. Lunge poses have a simultaneously powerful and grounding effect. The second one pictured above involves a forward fold, and arms placed on the floor. This may be modified – made simpler – by placing hands on the floor either side of the front foot, with arms straight.

7. Pyramid Pose

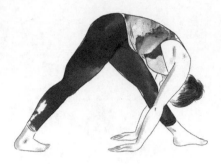

Benefit

This forward folding pose provides a deep hamstring stretch that brings freedom to the lower back and hips, while the forward bend also stimulates a free and even breath. Do this pose with blocks under your hands or something that gives you a little extra height if you have tighter hamstrings.

8. Extended Side Angle with Twist

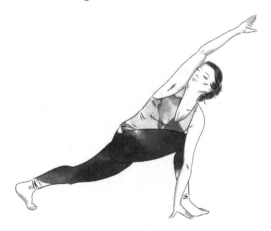

Benefit

This pose increases strength in the gluteal muscles, especially on the front leg, and use your abdominal muscles for stability. This calls on your strength and concentration. The added twist helps you learn to stabilize your body and hold with focus as your back muscles and shoulders open, and your abdomen tones. This brings your heart rate up as you concentrate and breathe, helping your nervous system get into condition, handling a little stress without straining.

9. One-Leg Downward-Facing Dog (to Counterpose Twists)

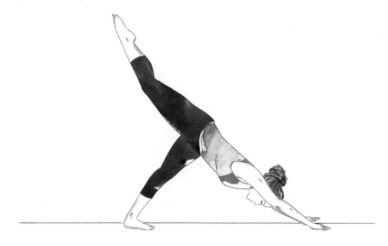

Benefit

This pose stretches out the back muscles evenly after a twist and focuses back at centre while you regulate your breath. After the standing twists, it's important to re-lengthen out through your hamstrings.

10. Pigeon Hip Stretch

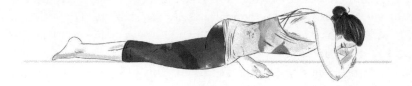

Benefit

This deep hip stretch can be very relaxing to the nervous system, and the forward-bending action turns the mind inward easily. It releases tension from the lower back by lengthening and releasing the piriformis, gluteal and adductor muscles.

11. Little Bridge Pose – Setubandha

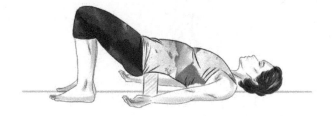

Benefit

This pose shows up in different forms – some of which are more relaxing and others more energizing. Here, it opens the breath into the chest, stretches the pectoral muscles, opens the diaphragm and lengthens the often-contracted belly muscles. This also brings circulation into the throat, where the thyroid and parathyroid reside. These two glands are associated with hormonal regulation, including digestion and sleep. This variation lifts the hips to the same height as the knees, which moves into a deeper curl in the upper back, stimulating the thoracic plexus of nerves and intensifying the energizing quality of the pose.

12. Seated Side Twist

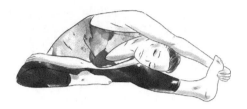

Benefit

This pose gives another form of back stretch and side stretch, while opening the hips and hamstrings. It is both grounding and energizing at the same time.

13. Sukhasana (Easy Pose)

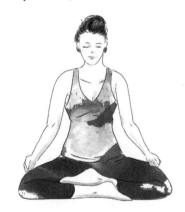

Benefit

A centring seated posture, which enables you to breathe evenly and fully into your lungs. It's stable as a seat, and lets you do some simple breath practices. This is a traditional meditation pose.

ADVANCED ASANA MORNING WAKE-UP

For those better acquainted with a yoga practice, the following suggestions may be useful for morning wake-up practices. They are not depicted here as their instruction relies on a competent and skilled teacher, and prior knowledge of yoga. They are available on the Super Sleep Yoga online course where they are demonstrated visually. However, these are guidelines to inspire practice, and creativity is encouraged.

1. Sun Salutations

2. Chair Pose

3. Downward-Facing Dog Splits

4. Sphinx Pose or Upward-Facing Dog

5. Forward-Facing Closed Prayer Twist

6. Side-Facing Warrior/Side Angle/Reverse Side-Facing Warrior Sequence

7. Virasana Variation

8. Navasana Variations

9. Pigeon Variations

10. Bridge/Wheel Pose

11. L-Shaped (Pre-Handstand) Pose at the Wall

12. Extended Child's Pose

13. Janu Sirsasana (Head to Knee Pose)/Side Stretch

14. Baddha Konasana (Diamond Pose)

15. Savasana

1. Sun Salutations

Benefit

Sun salutations can slightly elevate your heart rate, depending on how quickly or slowly you do them, while stretching and strengthening the major muscle groups of the body.

2. Chair Pose

Benefit

Chair is a strengthening pose, working the calf, thigh and gluteal muscles. It promotes concentration, balance and stability, enlivening your legs and raising your heart rate. When you sit low enough to engage your thighs strongly, you'll feel a fiery sensation. The pose fires you up and gets you ready for your day.

3. Downward-Facing Dog Splits

Benefit

A downward dog 'split' lengthens the belly and opens up the chest while stretching the hamstrings.

4. Sphinx Pose or Upward-Facing Dog

Sphinx Benefit

This pose lengthens the abdominal muscles and unhooks tension in the diaphragm, one of the most important breathing muscles. The upper back bend is energizing and helps to free your breath. When done with very strong engagement of the pelvic floor and front of the belly, this also creates more internal stability in the body.

Upward-Facing Dog Benefit

Upward-Facing Dog asks you to use your arm and shoulder muscles evenly, and encourages you to curl your shoulders back to open the chest. Lifting your legs off the floor means you need to engage your front belly muscles and pelvic floor deeply, to protect your lower back.

5. Forward-Facing Closed Prayer Twist

Benefit

This pose cultivates strength in the legs and hips. This version moves from an Invisible Chair (Uttkatasana) to the Standing Prayer Twist by twisting across the Chair Pose, and stepping a foot back. You need to use your gluteal muscles strongly as well as your calves and abdominals. This provides stability while you twist your torso, lengthening your back muscles and pressing your shoulders back, which both opens and activates the shoulders.

6. Side-Facing Warrior/Side Angle/Reverse Side-Facing Warrior Sequence

Benefit

This sequence (also known as Warrior II) cultivates strength and stability in the legs, while opening up the ribcage and lengthening the torso. A very enlivening combination!

7. Virasana Variation

Benefit

This pose is mid-way between virasana (Hero Pose) and ustrasana (Camel Pose). This variation strengthens the legs, by squeezing them to the centre, and activates the upper back and opens the chest, lengthening the abdominal muscles.

8. Navasana Variations

Benefit

Navasana or Boat Pose strengthens the abdominal muscles and creates full-body strength and integration. It is good for building stamina and stability.

9. Pigeon Variations

Benefit

A deep and grounding hip and gluteal stretch with variations that also open and release the thigh muscles.

10. Bridge/Wheel Pose
Benefit

This pose opens the chest, stretches the pectoral muscles, opens the diaphragm and lengthens the often-contracted belly muscles. This also brings circulation into the throat, where the thyroid and parathyroid reside. These two glands are associated with hormonal regulation, including digestion and sleep.

11. L-Shaped (Pre-Handstand) Pose at the Wall
Benefit

This pose is an excellent strengthener and energizer. The inversion brings a flush to your face, brings circulation into the lungs, and activates your arms.

12. Extended Child's Pose
Benefit

This pose is gently restorative, calming the body and mind whilst lengthening the muscles that line the spine and stretching the backs of the hips.

13. Janu Sirsasana (Head to Knee Pose)/Side Stretch
Benefit

This pose is an excellent counterpose to the leg strengtheners at the start of this series, with a deep hamstring stretch. The upper body here lengthens again, counterposing any compression that may have happened in your handstand preparation. The pose is calming and cooling, and releases the major muscle chains.

14. Baddha Konasana (Diamond Pose)
Benefit

This pose deeply stretches the outer hips and releases the chains of muscles up both sides of the spine. The forward-bending action is calming to the nervous system.

15. Savasana

Benefit

This is the great integration pose. It allows your body's circulation to rebalance. Also, this serves as training for your body and brain to learn the gentle art of relaxing into stillness: perfect practice for the pre-sleep moments.

Chapter Two

Energy Recovery for Better Sleep

The Nervous System and Breath

Wired or Tired? Energy Management, Prana Problems and Sleep

Prana is a concept that refers to the movement of vital life force. Other traditions call this Chi or Qi. People with sleep problems often complain of low energy and exhaustion, and about being 'wired' – and frequently swing between the two states. The lethargic low-energy situation leaves us feeling dragged down: we have difficulty with motivation, concentration or accomplishing things because there's not enough fuel to get there. For those feeling wired, being 'keyed up' may make it impossible to sit still, commit things to memory, settle down to rest, or respond to situations without reactivity. Both lead to an inability to achieve deep and restful sleep. People with long-term sleep problems often report feeling exhausted all day but getting a second wind at night, just at the time when they *should* be sleeping. This leads to a vicious cycle of exhaustion and frenetic energy. Sleep recovery is strengthened by managing our energy well throughout the day.

As we've seen in this book, human beings don't just have two states: on and off. Instead, we have energetic cycles throughout the day: at different times of the day it's natural to feel more alert or more lethargic. When we are aware of these cycles, we can work with them rather than fighting against them, which helps us to repair the mechanisms of sleep and wakefulness. By looking at the different dosha types, or constitutions (in the Introduction), we see that people have different energetic tendencies, and we can tailor our approach accordingly, giving the right practices for the person and time of day.

The more energetically 'grounding' practices are needed before sleep or during a middle-of-the-night wake-up. They tend to be calming and settling. They slow the heart rate and bring circulation downward in the body. The eyes and face will appear more relaxed and the muscles around the eyes will soften. By contrast, energetically elevating or 'activating' practices are needed to support wakefulness in the morning and at vital times throughout the day. These tend to bring more circulation into the upper body, raising the heart rate and causing a person to look brighter and more focused.

Over time, if your clients or students are practising the asana and breath practices in this programme, you will notice a difference in:

- how they hold their bodies (tense or more relaxed, exhausted or alert)

- how they breathe (faster or slower, broader or tighter)

- the expression on their faces (tense or relaxed, exhausted or focused)

- their pace of speech (more rapid or slower).

These are all cues to a person's energetic condition – clues about the state of their nervous system. Deeper healing of the sleep mechanisms – and the repatterning of the nervous system – starts when the client begins to come into their body by practising the Simple Sleep Sequence. Learning about the role of the breath and breathing to better manage energy then deepen the process, accelerating the results.

In this chapter, we look at the key elements that help re-establish the capacity to manage energy effectively; then we look at yogic and scientifically based ways of understanding the management of energy. We will discuss *how*, *why* and *when* the practices found at the end of this chapter work, so you can feel confident in choosing practices that are likely to help you or your clients. This will enable you to educate your students or clients about *why* they should practise the techniques you choose for them. Some will respond to the yogic explanations, others the scientific.

This chapter introduces:

- yogic approaches to energy: the Doshas and Vayus

- how the nervous system works, and particularly how breath influences it

- practices that help recondition your ability to sleep and rest easily:

  - calming breath practices that help to recover the capacity to 'ground' energy

  - energizing breath practices that foster sustainable alertness.

The Five Pranas: The Movement of Life Force, Grounding and Energizing

Generations ago, yoga practitioners began to sense and categorize, based on their own observations of subtle sensation, how circulation and 'energy' move within the body. If we are to help people to repair their mechanisms of relaxation and sleep holistically, this understanding can help. The concept of the five prana vayus as explained in the yogic texts called the Vedas (Feuerstein, 2011; Frawley, 2013) refer to the five directions of lifeforce or 'winds'. We can understand intuitively that our inhalation and exhalation affect us differently. When we move or remain still, we experience differences in our energetic state. We can also feel blocked or over-stimulated generally, or notice how some areas are more blocked while others are highly charged up. The following is summarized in Feuerstein (2011).

1. Prana – the incoming and rising current of the life force connected with the inhalation and with the heart region and the head.

2. Apana, the descending current, associated with exhalation and with the navel and lower abdomen.

3. Udana, the rising current located in the throat and associated with speech, expelling air (belching!) and other similar functions.

4. Samana, the midcurrent located in the abdomen and chiefly responsible for digestion.

5. Vyana, the diffuse current pervading the entire body that functions, even in the absence of inhalation and exhalation.

Sleep and the Pranas

The two most important of these, for our purposes, relate to the inhalation (prana) and exhalation (apana). We make use of these 'rising' and 'descending' qualities in our therapeutic understanding of movements and breath practices that help us to get 'down' to sleep or get 'up' in the morning. Apana and prana vayus correspond to the main types of asana and breath practices we use to recover sleep and heal insomnia.

In the sleep and wake time yoga sequences, we seek to balance the circulation and 'pranas' of the entire body, for a sense of evenness. No one body part or area is emphasized to the exclusion of others. However, depending on the desired effect (grounding or energizing), the sequences do focus more heavily on certain areas. The Simple Sleep Sequence and Deeper Sleep Sequence address the entire body, but favour the movement of circulation downward into the legs, lower belly and hips. This stimulates apana vayu, which is settling in nature. Gently lengthening the exhalation increases the grounding effect. Through our modern neurophysiological understanding, we understand how the practices stimulate the parasympathetic nervous system, which will be discussed in greater detail below.

Morning wake-up practices, by contrast, bring breath, movement and circulation upward towards the heart and upper parts of the lungs, with vigorous arm movements that open the body and inversions which place the head below the heart, bringing circulation to the face. These are done with the 'stronger' form of ujjayii breath – which tends to be more heating and stimulating. These practices activate the sympathetic nervous system.

Daily Energy: An Ayurvedic Perspective

Earlier in this book we explored the Ayurvedic doshas as they correspond to different body–mind constitutions. The Ayurvedic system also tracks the ways in which prana moves throughout the day, noting that different times of day have different energetic qualities and relate to different bodily functions. The yoga practitioners based their understanding on observations of human beings, animals and plants and how they responded to different times of day – in the context of light and dark patterns. This presaged our modern understanding of circadian rhythms, and saw these energies in terms of the doshas that predominate and their qualities. Aligning with these natural rhythms means we can manage and tailor daily habits accordingly, promoting harmony within ourselves and with nature. The times may shift slightly forward or back depending upon the season and your geographic location, but it's useful to notice the pattern and how energy differs throughout the day (Frawley, 2013).

Kapha: 6am–10am and 6pm–10pm

This dosha is associated most strongly with the earth element, and is the most stable of all three energies. It is said that our deepest habits are established during the kapha hours – at the start and end of the day. According to Ayurvedic guidelines, if it's difficult to wake up in this time horizon, it may actually be easier to awaken before 6am.

Ayurvedic sources state that exercise done in the kapha hours stands the best chance of developing into a lasting habit. The morning kapha hours are ideal, with the evening hours being the next best alternative. Very vigorous exercise is best kept to the earlier evening kapha hours so that body temperature and hormones may move towards sleep properly.

Many people establish poor habits by delaying sleep past kapha time, and into pitta time. When we begin to notice our true energy patterns, we may notice that, unhindered by caffeine or other stimulants, we are naturally sleepy for the first time as it gets dark. This strong urge towards sleep in the early evening after it has become dark is the pull of the kapha energy. Many people over-ride the sleep urge and stay up into pitta time, which accounts for the 'second wind' they experience, and difficulties sleeping later.

During the kapha hours, this programme recommends:

- morning sleep 'mop-up' or energizing asana practice, and energizing pranayama practice, between 6am and 10am

- evening sleep sequences between 6pm and 10pm (close to bedtime) with calming, settling breath practice.

Pitta: 10am–2pm and 10pm–2am

The pitta or fire energy facilitates our ability to concentrate. We are most focused and alert during the pitta times of the day. Pitta is associated with the processes of digestion and appetite. Ayurveda teaches that it is best to eat your biggest meal of the day at lunch, when it can be most effectively digested during waking hours. If we are awake into pitta time at night, the digestive processes active during that time can cause us to reach for midnight snacks – another good reason to be asleep before 10pm. If we stay awake too late, digestion kicks in and causes us to feel hungry.

Generally, between 10am and 2pm is the time for work or other activities, as well as eating a mid-day meal.

Vata: 2pm–6pm and 2am–6am

Vata is the least stable of the three energies and the most expansive. When it is dominant, during the afternoon and during the time you are, I hope, asleep, it is difficult to establish routine. In the afternoon in particular, we may be prone to changeable moods and impulsiveness as our energy dissipates. However, this energy promotes creativity and imagination. We may be better able to learn new things or focus on creative thinking during the vata times of day.

When we get to sleep early enough, we are in the deeper dream state during the last part of sleep, when vata dosha predominates. Its expansive nature relates to the nature of late-night dreaming. If we are able to get to sleep in the kapha time, and do the bodily restoration sleep and digestive processing during the pitta hours, we get to vata time in our deep sleep and reap the benefits.

The afternoon is a great time for mind-managing mid-afternoon meditation or a restorative power-down. Those with sleep difficulties often experience a crash in energy around 2pm. Instead of reaching for caffeine or stressing out to press through the exhaustion, this is the time for a mid-day power-down that sparks sustainable energy.

Understanding the Body–Brain–
Breath–Sleep Connection
An Over-Activated Nervous System Epidemic

The sleeplessness epidemic seems to be worsening, and far greater numbers of people are reporting delayed, interrupted or poor-quality sleep. This is no surprise when we look at the modern pace of life and the rate at which the human brain is asked to process information and respond to stimuli. Constantly plugged in, many of us are online most of the day with laptops and smartphones. News stories can 'break' at any time of day, and can be emailed to you directly, whether you are lying in bed awake in the middle of the night or on a secluded beach on an idyllic island. Information reaches us everywhere and, as soon as we switch on our devices, there is no insulation from any news – personal or global. We may have a stress response to incoming information at any time of day. Every time this happens, it can stimulate the release of the stress hormones cortisol and/or adrenaline. Growing evidence suggests that social media can create a mini-boost of dopamine to which we may become addicted, just like any dopamine-spiking process or substance. We are more subject to intrusion, more likely to seek external stimulation and less likely to allow the nervous system to settle than ever before.

As we will see in this chapter, heart rate corresponds with breath rate, signalling agitation or relaxation. A comparison of how we breathe now with how our great-grandparents breathed a century ago is rather staggering. In the 1920s, anatomy texts cited that the average adult took about eight to ten breaths per minute, but 100 years later, after the digital revolution, even the most relaxed among us take about 12 breaths per minute. Essentially, if our breathing is faster, then our nervous systems are in a heightened state of low-grade fight-or-flight. It's no wonder that problems of anxiety, insomnia and sleeplessness are on the rise.

One of our top jobs as therapists and healers, doctors and teachers is to harness the potential to repattern and recondition the responses of the human nervous system so that we can sleep again. In this chapter, you'll see how breath directly affects the two branches of the autonomic nervous system that are responsible for the stress response and the relaxation response. The practices in this chapter are carefully designed and time-tested. They have immediate effects and have great promise, when practised over time, of creating real and lasting change towards a healthier pattern of sleep and waking.

Yoga for Sleep: Neurophysiology

We turn now to some nervous system basics. The summary of the nervous system was generously contributed by Heather Mason of the Minded Institute, with whom I offered continuing professional development courses for several years. As a researcher, Heather offered some possible underlying neurophysiological reasons why the practices, which I have used successfully in clinical practice for years, work.

You may be very well acquainted with the neurophysiology, you may be exposed to this information for the first time, or somewhere in between. In this section, the intention is to strike a balance – without disappearing into too much detail, I seek to give you the practice-relevant basics.

The Nervous System: An Overview

Your nervous system consists of two major parts:

- The central nervous system is made up of the brain and spinal cord.

- The peripheral nervous system links the brain and spinal cord with your organs, muscles, bones and viscera. We can think of it as the body-to-brain messaging system.

The figure on the next page shows how it's all connected.

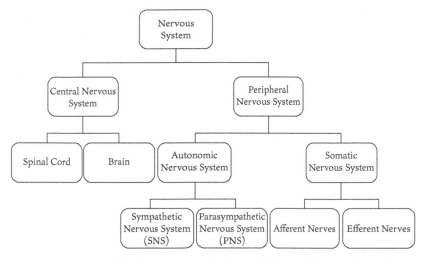

A Map of the Nervous System (courtesy of The Minded Institute)

The peripheral nervous system sends and receives signals from the organs and limbs. This lets the body and brain communicate and share information. This peripheral nervous system has two branches:

- The somatic nervous system includes the muscles and the motor and sensory neurons.

- The autonomic nervous system (ANS) deals with activation and relaxation through changes in nervous system response. The ANS maintains our equilibrium by adjusting physiological responses to maintain constant balance in the nervous system and respond to the environment in appropriate nervous-system ways. The ANS increases or decreases our heart rate, stimulates or inhibits digestion, quickens or slows breathing, and regulates salivation, perspiration, sexual arousal, urination, blood flow to muscles and organs, and the contraction and relaxation of smooth muscle (including that which lines the blood vessels).

The ANS uses many feedback loops to convey information from our senses – from both the body and the environment – back to the brain. Different parts of the brain then organize responses. For example, when we are in danger, the ANS organizes the physical response of increased blood pressure, working with other parts of the brain to provoke the fear response and a cascade of other processes that also include the release of stress hormones through the endocrine system.

Mostly, we don't notice the autonomic nervous system doing its job. We can't really tell when our digestion is speeding up. However, this part of the nervous system is unique in that we do have *partial control* over it. This means that we can directly influence the ANS to reduce stress, improve the quality of our sleep, and feel more awake during the day. Yoga practices including stretches and regulation of the breath can influence the autonomic system, changing your physical conditions and emotional responses immediately and powerfully.

The ANS has two branches that work together like a see-saw. The sympathetic nervous system is the part that 'activates', and the parasympathetic nervous system is the part which 'relaxes'. When one is heightened, the other is less active. The one that's dominant depends on our internal and external environments.

The Sympathetic Nervous System: Fight/Flight Activation

The sympathetic nervous system (SNS) excites and activates the brain and body, mobilizing it for action. The effects of SNS activity are most apparent under conditions of stress, excitement or fear and are classically referred to, at the extreme end of stimulation, as the 'fight or flight' response. When we are in a sympathetic-dominant mode, the following happens:

- Heart rate increases and more blood flows to the muscles and the brain to prepare for action. Remember, blood brings oxygen to cells, which is vital for cells to function.

- Blood flow is diverted away from the digestive and sexual organs as survival-based processes need to take over.

- Blood is shunted away from the skin, so that if we are wounded, we do not lose too much blood.

- Respiratory rate increases so that oxygen can be rapidly transported around the body.

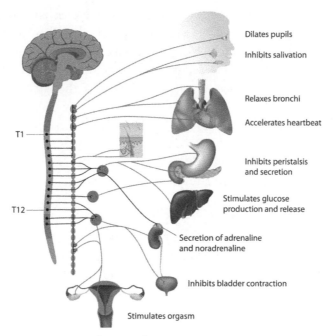

Dilates pupils

Inhibits salivation

Relaxes bronchi

Accelerates heartbeat

T1

Inhibits peristalsis
and secretion

Stimulates glucose
production and release

T12

Secretion of adrenaline
and noradrenaline

Inhibits bladder contraction

Stimulates orgasm

The Sympathetic Nervous System

When the SNS is in full-blown response mode, it gears up the body and brain for a response to whatever is causing the fear, stress and/or excitement, enabling the individual to be totally focused on that stimulus. The SNS is a catabolic system, meaning that it breaks down energy in the body. Energy is used to prepare us for defence or action. In less threatening circumstances we draw on the SNS to mobilize our energy to get from place to place, meet deadlines, attend to responsibilities and have an active life. Some sympathetic drive is necessary. It provides us with a basic ability to respond and mobilize energy when needed or to cope with an actual physical threat.

Unfortunately, we over-use the SNS. We have not adapted to the low-level stresses that we face every day – the emotional response to a threat to one's job can feel as life threatening as being chased by a tiger. Chronic SNS over-activation can leave the body and mind exhausted as it uses up energy and depletes the body's resources; remember it's catabolic, it breaks things down. Furthermore, we are not often able to respond to sympathetic arousal in ways that the body is programmed to do. The rapid heartbeat, blood to muscles, etc. are all preparing us to spring into action, which in the modern world we often do not do. When humans were hunter-gatherers, the fight or flight response was an advantageous strategy that kept us safe over and over again: see the tiger, sense the fear, run to safety. Those with hyper-sensitive stress responses were more likely to survive. Many modern problems can't be solved by running away or fighting. Most social and financial problems require rational thought and calm, rather than panic and physical mobilization.

Unfortunately, the responses of the SNS in these situations only serve to make our life more difficult and decrease our chances of survival. Additionally, today's constant and daily stressors lead to a continual activation of the stress response. However, in these situations, summoning energy and capabilities to take physical action isn't what's required and so we're left feeling fearful and hyper-aroused. When fight or flight are neither necessary nor possible, and the activation response has become overly sensitive, yoga and breath practices can provide a vital resource for mitigating the stress response and reconditioning a right-sized response to stress or perceived threat.

The Parasympathetic Nervous System: Rest and Digest

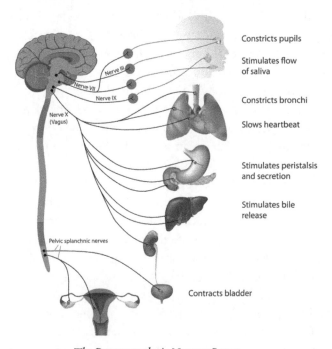

The Parasympathetic Nervous System

The parasympathetic nervous system (PNS) acts as a counterbalance to the sympathetic nervous system – it is dominant when we are resting and sleeping or when our digestive processes are active. During these periods, the PNS:

- reduces heart rate

- provides blood flow all over the body and is less selective than sympathetic response

- dilates blood vessels, leading to the digestive tract increasing blood flow to aid digestion

- stimulates digestion and accelerates peristalsis

- stimulates the immune system and the building of immune cells.

In contrast to the SNS, the PNS is *anabolic* in nature. It rebuilds the body's resources. The PNS is the default in a healthy human being, with the SNS ramping up and dampening its activity as and when required.

While the PNS should be the dominant mode when we are at rest, as a society we are experiencing a neurophysiological shift towards greater SNS arousal, as more of the population lives faster, consumes more caffeine and other stimulants and is more highly susceptible to agitation through the continual input of information than in any generation before. If we are in sympathetic mode too often, we are likely to feel extremely fatigued, but paradoxically this type of exhaustion makes it harder to drop into parasympathetic mode, making more elusive the sleep we so desperately need.

The Relaxation Response: A Key to Healing

In order to recondition our capacity to sleep, we need to redevelop the ability to relax fully and deeply. Herbert Benson, a cardiologist at Harvard Medical School and a pioneer in the field of mind–body medicine, found that the body can enter a deep parasympathetic state where it uses less oxygen and glucose (meaning we use less energy) than at any other time, including during sleep. He termed this state the 'relaxation response'. His research shows it takes a minimum of three minutes to enter this state, although usually it's longer. For those struggling with fatigue and insomnia, it is essential to learn how to enter this relaxation-based state to allow the body to recalibrate and start conserving and rebuilding resources that are depleted when sleep is poor or lacking.

I explain this process to my clients as 'putting energy back on the grid' when we are tired. Spending time moving into the relaxation response re-trains the body and brain in the states needed to move towards sleep, and to stay asleep.

Managing Stress and Relaxation: Breath and the Vagus Nerve

With this information about the SNS and PNS in mind, we return to the key fact: we can influence our stress and relaxation responses directly. In fact, how you breathe changes your mind and sense of self. The information here, about the role of the vagus nerve, is drawn from an article by Heather Mason (2017).

Since 2005, integrative psychiatrists Patricia Gerbarg and Richard Brown (Brown and Gerbarg, 2012; Gerbarg and Brown, 2005) have looked at how regular pranayama practice alters specific neurophysiological pathways, spurring changes in how we think and feel. In conjunction with psychiatrist and neurologist Chris Streeter, they offer explanations for how breathing practices alter our sense of self through changes in the brain (called neuroplasticity). They draw on Dr Stephen Porges' research about the vagus nerve (the major parasympathetic nerve) and Dr Budd Craig's findings on the insula cortex, a deep structure in the brain associated with our sense of body image, feeling and self. Their research suggests that the vagus nerve, which runs through much of the respiratory tract, picks up on our breath's rate, intensity and steadiness (or lack thereof) and sends this information to the brain stem, which passes the message through neurons to limbic structures which encode our instinctual and emotional responses. Lastly, it passes this breath information on to the frontal lobe of the brain, which governs our rational thought and our capacity to reassess our experience. In this way the vagus nerve picks up breath information and tells the brain about our state – relaxed or stressed. Thus, when we breathe more deeply and slowly we can send the message from the body to the brain that we are safe and can relax and release tension.

According to Streeter and Gerberg's hypothesis, slow and controlled breath stimulates the thalamus to release a major anti-anxiety neurotransmitter called GABA, which promotes a greater sense of calm and ease (Streeter, Gerberg and Saper, 2012). The GABA release suppresses the limbic system's fear response, and increases activity in frontal brain structures and the insula, which let us think more clearly. So when we breathe slowly and deeply, we increase the anti-anxiety neurotransmitter that helps us to feel calmer and overcome fear.

Changing Your Breathing: Shifting Your Body and Brain Responses

Inhaling or Exhaling: Stimulating versus Relaxing

The simplest of things can make a tremendous difference to how we feel and how our bodies and minds respond to our internal and external worlds. When we exhale, our heart rate is slightly less rapid than it is when we inhale. When we exhale, via messaging through the vagus nerve, the heart rate is slightly inhibited. We can effectively slow our heart rate by breathing out for longer than we inhale. In terms of yoga therapy for insomnia, when we help our students and clients to breathe with this awareness, they have at their disposal a simple way to calm the nervous system and quell stress responses all day long, as well as in the run-up to sleep. The lengthened exhale is a key feature of sleep-focused yoga sequences for this reason. When we seek to energize, we seek to gently stimulate the sympathetic nervous system. Lengthening the inhale relative to the exhale is a way to achieve this effect.

Fast versus Slow Breath: Lung 'Stretch Fibres' that Stimulate or Relax

Our lungs are equipped with sensors that detect changes in the depth and pace of our breath. Slow breathing activates slow-adapting pulmonic (lung) stretch fibres (SARs) in our lungs, which send a calming message from the body to the brain. Slow, rhythmic breathing indicates that the body is in a relaxed state and the brain begins to respond with the neurochemistry of relaxation. On the other hand, when we breathe rapidly, the rapidly adapting pulmonic stretch fibres

(RARs) fire, and the brain receives the message to kick into a higher level of activation. Learning to slow down and deepen the breath is the key to accessing a more relaxed state.

Breath and the Nadis: Stimulating and Relaxing

The ancient yogis have long known something that modern science has confirmed through research (Shannahoff-Khalsa, 2006): that the sympathetic nervous system is stimulated by breath in and out of the right nostril, and the parasympathetic nervous system is stimulated by breath in and out of the left nostril. The yogis associated different energetic channels with the left (the ida nadi) and the right (the pingala nadi) and related them to the qualities of moon (relaxation) and sun (activation) respectively. Knowing this, those who have enough ease with breathing and some control over their breath may use their breath accordingly and adjust their level of activation or relaxation.

Keeping the Breathing Simple: Rationale for Practices

In this programme, I keep the breath practices, or pranayama, very simple, because I want everyone to be able to access the benefits, whether they are seasoned yogis or have never considered yoga before. I want the majority of people to be able to do their practices anywhere and without strain. I have chosen to take breath-count practices out of this programme for the simple reason that most people find them difficult if they have never worked with their breath before, or have never practised yoga.

Intermediate and Kundalini Methods: Breath Retention and Counts

There are some practices that I could never have benefited from as a new yoga practitioner – the ones that require counting the beats of an inhale, holding the breath, and counting the beats of an exhale. I still consider these intermediate pranayama, since for many beginners they can be rather difficult. I found it very stressful keeping count, and also as both an asthmatic at that time, and a trauma survivor, breath retention of any kind was too panic-inducing. Practices that involve breath retention and counting may be highly valuable to people who are either able to do them immediately or are willing to undergo a bit of discomfort in learning them. These include Shabad Kriya, a Kundalini breath and mantra technique, and 4:7:8 breath (a technique that involves inhaling for a count of four, holding the breath for a count of seven, and then exhaling for a count of eight).

One of the strongest proponents of these techniques is the highly respected Harvard-based sleep researcher and Kundalini yogi Sat Bir Khalsa (with whom I have co-authored a yoga therapy for insomnia chapter, in Mason and Birch (2018), as mentioned above). As Dr Khalsa's research shows, for some people these techniques work well and powerfully. I don't often include them in my work with beginning students and clients because (a) this programme is not based in the Kundalini yoga methodology as my own experience of it is minimal, but instead draws on a Hatha yoga perspective, and (b) my clinical experience and teaching experience have shown me that the barriers to beginning with these practices *may* be too high for many people who are in acute distress and who are not sleeping well. They may, however, be welcome practices as breath and attention develop.

The text below brings together an understanding of the doshic approach aligned with the daily circadian rhythms, with practices that develop the grounding (apana) and energizing (prana) needed to restore balance to the nervous system. Yogic techniques like pranayama and marma points, when done at the most advantageous times of day, aid the recovery of the sleep and wake mechanisms needed to get better, more rewarding rest with sustainable energy all day.

The Practices: Daily Energy Recovery

Each of the practices below has the power to shift a person's physical and psychological states immediately and to create a lasting benefit in terms of reconditioning the nervous system – and its ability to respond appropriately by activating and relaxing as needed – in the longer term. First, we examine what those with sleep difficulties may need across the span of a day and then outline which practices are more beneficial at different times.

Morning Restoration and Wake-Up

It's reasonable that too little – or unsatisfying – sleep will leave us feeling tired in the morning. If this is ongoing, the feeling may move towards desperate exhaustion. It may seem counterintuitive, but one of the best methods for dealing with morning exhaustion is not to try to sleep an extra few minutes in bed, but to get out of bed, do some gentle movement and settle into specifically designed restorative poses that 'put some energy back on the grid'.

One or more of the restorative yoga poses in this book can be incredibly valuable for enabling a person to face the day. Ranging from a single posture held for up to 15 minutes, to three or four postures that comprise a practice of up to an hour, a restorative practice can promote greater calm and better, more sustainable energy. I call this 'mopping up after a bad night's sleep' – it is a basic tool for sustainable, holistic insomnia recovery. This early in the day, it doesn't interfere with the homeostatic (body balancing) drive to sleep but prevents the person from being in a heightened yet depleted state, and makes it possible to draw energy from rest rather than caffeine or stress hormones.

After putting some rest into the system, I recommend catalysing the awakening response with strong breath practices designed to bring in more oxygen and activate the body-to-brain wake-up cues. This, in conjunction with 'layering in rest' throughout the duration of the day, ensures that the body and mind are not continually running on empty, in exhausted sympathetic nervous system mode.

Power-Down Breaths During the Day: Putting Energy Back on the Grid

As we've seen, it's vitally important to decrease the stress response in order to recondition the nervous system in ways that promote better balance and deeper rest. Using the calming breath practices enables us to layer in the nervous system balancing effects throughout the day. Resting in specific ways throughout the day gives us the opportunity to enact the relaxation response, entering the parasympathetic-dominant mode. This has the immediate effect of putting energy back on the grid, and the longer-term effect of retraining your body and brain in the important art of relaxation.

I'm not a big fan of machine metaphors when it comes to our bodies and our sleep, but someone once used an example that I thought was helpful: a factory can produce goods 24 hours a day, but if the machinery gets too hot and if you don't let it cool down, then even machines start to break down. Rest times are our way of cooling down our physical and mental processing during the day. Most people, though their machinery is over-heated, will keep going, over-riding the afternoon slump or sense of exhaustion by consuming caffeine or just pushing through. This is like asking an over-heated machine to work harder. Little wonder that at times those who push through the need to rest become ill, experiencing physical or psychological strain.

Sleep Time Power-Down Practices

The majority of the practices in this programme are designed to power-down the nervous system. They are best used when there is a need to lower the heart rate, decrease stress responses, and to condition the response to being in the bedroom at night. Those who have had difficulty sleeping can find it very valuable to breathe easily and freely in the bedroom, de-coupling the bedroom from feelings of anxiety and experiencing more pleasant sensations in real time. As with all practices, there are immediate and longer-term benefits. For those who suffer from anxiety, hyper-arousal, emotional strain or breathing difficulties, the practices work in the short term and, as with all yoga practices, create greater resilience in the long term. The simple, effective breath practices in this programme radically alter the experience of getting to sleep at night, getting back to sleep if there are middle-of-the-night wake-ups, or resting when needed to restore energy.

CALMING AND SLEEP-INDUCING BREATH PRACTICES

1. Ujjayii Breath

Ujjayii is referred to as the classic 'yoga breath'. It creates a sense of balance and makes all the poses more effective. If you were to try the same postures and stretches both with and without the ujjayii breath, you would probably feel that postures made less of an impact on you if you weren't using this simple and powerful regulating breath. When I teach the Simple Sleep Sequence in my courses, I ask students to report back how they feel at the end. If there's a student who doesn't feel more relaxed at the end of the sequence, I make sure that they are able to do the ujjayii breath along with the movements, and the poses begin to work perfectly. This breath combines with the movement almost magically.

Ujjayii breath produces a sound like ocean waves in the distance, caused by a gentle constriction in the back of the throat – a toning of the glottis. This breath focuses the mind on the sound of breath and, when done with even inhalation, has a 'balancing' effect. An elongated exhale, or a longer count on the out-breath, tends to calm the nervous system more effectively.

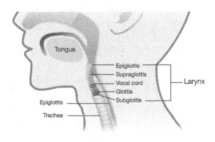

The Larynx

There are many different instructions about this breath with varied effects. The common components are:

- breathing in and out through the nose only (mouth closed)

- an intentional constriction at the back of the throat that regulates the flow of breath

- a hissing sound often likened to the sound of ocean waves.

Step by Step

- Bring your palm a few inches from your face.

- Inhale and then exhale through the mouth like you would to fog a mirror, feeling the breath on your palm.

- This demonstrates the flow of breath while toning the glottis at the back of the throat, which is an important part of the breath technique.

- Release your hand down to your lap.

- Now create the same tone in the back of your throat but exhale through the nose with the mouth closed. Ujjayii is done as a closed-mouth breath.

- For beginners, it is useful to start by inhaling normally through the nose with no tone in the back of the throat, and exhaling through the nose with a gentle constriction or 'hissing sound' in the back of the throat.

- Then, if comfortable, add the constriction and gentle hissing sound on inhale as well as exhale with an even breath-count, keeping the mouth closed.

Ujjayii Breath: Soft or Strong?

When ujjayii is done with bandhas (inner locks), as it is traditionally practised in Ashtanga yoga, breath is essentially forced upward and centralized in the upper chest. This has a heating and stimulating effect. This is consistent with Ashtanga's emphasis on *tapasya*, or spiritually transformative heat, as a guiding principle of asana practice. Breathing in this way may build capacity to manage more activated states in the longer term. However, in the short term, for people with anxiety disorders, trauma or highly agitated nervous systems, as we often see related to insomnia, it may feel 'over-heating' or support already well-entrenched nervous system over-activation.

Another way of performing the ujjayii breath – which is more helpful over time for the treatment of insomnia – is to maintain the features of nasal breathing, tone of the glottis and the gentle sound while 'filling' the lower back part of the lungs. This means directing attention into – and feeling as though you are 'filling' – the area of your back *below* the shoulders and *above* the sacrum. This is where the kidneys are located. Breathing in this way, keeping the ujjayii's throat constriction both subtle and gentle, tends to have the opposite effect to the strong ujjayii. Breath becomes softer and fuller.

While it is not possible to say that this breath 'cleanses' or technically balances adrenals, it is true that the adrenal glands sit atop the kidneys, and bringing circulation to an area may balance it energetically and physically. In practice, I have observed that breathing into the lower lungs has a powerful de-stressing, de-adrenalizing effect on the vast majority of my students and clients.

Follow these instructions to refine ujjayii breath for sleep – focusing down and back with the breath.

Step by Step

- Find a breath-count with a pace and timing that is easy and stress-free for you. If you gasp for breath or feel tightness, it's too intense and it's better to back off.

- To optimize ujjayii breath for sleep, focus on breathing into the lowest part of the back.

- Fill with breath (like you'd fill a glass of water) from the bottom to the top gently.

- This keeps the practitioner from focusing on the upper front third of the lungs, which tends to be more stimulating.

- Focusing down and back with the breath tends to be more calming.

- Repeat several times, refining and calming the breath, keeping the face, throat and jaw relaxed. When done, breathe gently and evenly through both nostrils a few times and then return to natural breath.

2. Three-Part Breath: Modified Dirga Pranayama

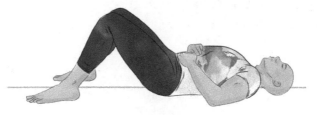

Low Belly Breath

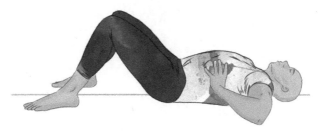

Middle Ribcage Breath

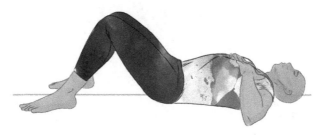

Upper Chest Breath

This exercise helps bring breath into the lungs, ribcage and torso evenly, fully and calmly. To relax and prepare for sleep, do this practice lying on the floor or bed with the soles of the feet on the floor and knees pointing upward. Keep a natural arch in the low back.

Postural note: do not press the lower back into the floor Pilates-style – this will contract the abdominals, inhibit the movement of the diaphragm and block the flow of breath.

Modification note: this breath practice may be done in a seated position where necessary.

Step by Step
Part 1 – Lower Abdomen (Sacrum, Intestines and Reproductive Organs)

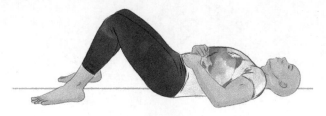

Low Belly Breath

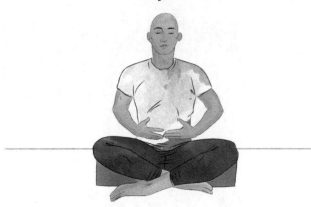

Seated Alternative for Low Belly Breath

- Place your hands on the front of your lower belly – beneath the belly button, inside the hip bones.

- When you breathe in, puff up your lower belly, letting the belly muscles stretch, and release to make a 'Buddha belly'.

- As you exhale, release the belly muscles, so they relax and flatten down – and your hands will descend.

- Notice the weight of the pelvic bones and lower back (sacrum) on the floor as you exhale.

- This improves circulation in the lower digestive area and relaxes the nerves around your lower back that affect digestion.

Part 2 – Middle Ribcage (Solar Plexus, Diaphragm and Stomach)

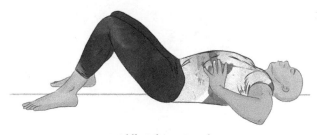

Middle Ribcage Breath

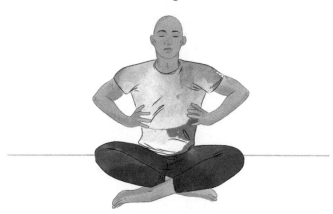

Seated Alternative for Middle Ribcage Breath

- Wrap your fingers around the front of your ribcage, with your thumbs around the sides pointing to the back.

- Place your index finger laterally across your ribcage at the bottom of the sternum (where the bra-line is for women). Keep your shoulders relaxed and elbows on the floor.

- As you inhale, inflate the front and back of your middle ribcage – and expand sideways at the same time. Breathe into the full space round your ribs, into the full circumference of the ribcage.

- As you exhale, your ribcage naturally narrows, and the muscles relax.

- This practice stretches and tones the diaphragm and moves the intercostal muscles, helping to relax and improve breathing.

Part 3 – Upper Chest (Top of Lungs, Shoulders and Neck)

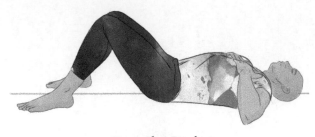

Upper Chest Breath

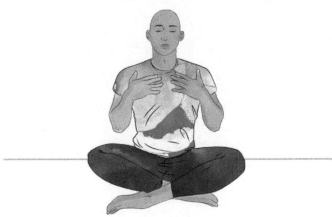

Seated Alternative for Upper Chest Breath

Often, we tense or lift the shoulders when breathing in, which helps lock stress into the body. It is important to de-couple the breath with the tensing of the shoulders, and learn to keep the shoulders and neck relaxed, as well as the face, staying relaxed on the in-breath.

- Place your hands above your chest, right below your collarbones, with your thumbs out towards your shoulders.

- As you inhale, breathe as though you could direct your breath into the back of your shoulders – keeping them relaxed.

- As you exhale, release the shoulders and upper chest into the floor, so your shoulder-blades and the back of your skull feel weightier and the muscles around them can release their grip.

ALL THREE TOGETHER: THE BREATH WAVE

- Inhale and expand first at the low belly, then take the breath up to the middle ribs, and finally to the upper chest in a wave-like fashion without strain.

- Exhale to release the breath from the top of the chest, through the middle ribs and downward towards the belly.

- You can use your hands to direct your attention to where you're breathing.

- Practise so that you can do this with awareness on each part separately and smoothly from bottom to top and top to bottom.

3. Alternate Nostril Breathing

This practice uses the physiology described earlier in this chapter – the left nostril's correspondence to the parasympathetic nervous system (lunar channel) and the right nostril's correspondence with the sympathetic nervous system (solar channel).

The basic practice involves breathing in and out for the same duration, called sama-vrtti (Sanskrit, meaning 'same wave'), and fosters balance between the two branches of the nervous system. Once a person is proficient in this practice, it's possible to manipulate the duration of inhale or exhale to achieve the desired effects. For example, lengthening the exhale will foster relaxation, while increasing the inhalation will be more stimulating.

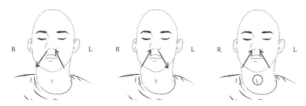

Nadi sodhana: inhale left, exhale right. Then inhale right, exhale left.

Balancing breath through both nostrils after any of the nostril breaths.

Alternate Nostril Breathing

Step by Step

- First, take the hand position called 'chin mudra' with your right hand. To do this:

  - Look at your right palm, then fold your index and middle fingers in toward your palm.

  - Tuck the tip of your thumb in to touch the tip of your ring finger, with your little finger right alongside your ring finger.

- Bring this towards your nose and separate the thumb and ring finger tips, so that you can balance the thumb tip on the right side of the bridge of your nose, and the ring finger on the left.

- Move your thumb and ring finger tips down to the space right where the fleshy bit of the nose joins the bony bit of the nose.

- Inhale through the left nostril while placing gentle pressure on the right side with your thumb.

- Breathe in to the top of the inhale without strain, and then pause for a moment.

- Then switch the finger pressure to the opposite side, so that you can breathe out through the right nostril.

- At the end of your exhale, again without straining or pressing the breath out forcefully, pause gently and begin the in-breath into the right nostril.

- When done, pause and exhale through the left nostril.

- This completes one 'round' with inhale and exhale through alternate nostrils.

- Begin a new round by inhaling through the left nostril and exhale right. Then inhale right and exhale left.

3a. Surya Bhadra and Chandra Bhedana

In addition, the practices of Surya Bhedana and Chandra Bhedana focus on breathing in and out through only one nostril, bringing the stimulation of the lunar/parasympathetic/relaxing channel or the solar/sympathetic/activating channel, respectively. This practice is best if you have no trouble breathing, as it isn't a practice you can do with acute asthma or nasal obstruction.

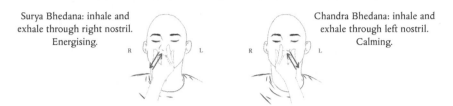

Surya Bhedana: inhale and exhale through right nostril. Energising.

Chandra Bhedana: inhale and exhale through left nostril. Calming.

Surya Bhedana and Chandra Bhedana

4. Kundalini Breath/Mantra for Sleep (Shabad Kriya)

This practice, from the Kundalini yoga tradition, combines breath with mantra. The full cycle of breath is done in 22 beats, first an inhalation for four counts while mentally reciting a mantra (Sa Ta Na Ma), then the breath is held for 16 counts mentally repeating the same mantra (Sa Ta Na Ma) four times, followed by a two-count exhale silently reciting a mantra (Wahe Guru). It's indicated as a pre-bedtime routine and can be done throughout the day. This practice has been subjected to clinical trials by the Harvard Medical School-based yoga researcher Sat Bir Khalsa, who details the Shabad Kriya practice in his book *Your Brain on Yoga* (Khalsa with Gould, 2012). In the studies, participants were instructed to practise this technique daily for eight weeks just before bedtime. Overall, Khalsa's research observed significant average improvements in both sleep duration and quality.

In my yoga therapy practice, I work with many people whose insomnia is related to trauma and hyper-arousal, and their capacity to perform breath retention is not immediately available. The practice may take them some time to build, and my own teaching and practice background is not primarily Kundalini based, so I don't often teach it. For those who are experienced with teaching Kundalini yoga, and have clients with the capacity and desire to work with the breath in this way, it can offer great benefits. It is said that if practised regularly, sleep will be deep and relaxed. After a few months, the rhythm of your breath as you sleep will be subconsciously regulated in rhythm with the mantra.

Step by Step

POSTURE AND EYES

- Sit in any comfortable posture with the spine elongated and the head upright. Place your hands in your lap, with your palms up, with the right hand over the left so that the thumb tips touch and point forward. Focus your eyes on the tip of your nose, with eyelids half-closed.

BREATH AND MANTRA

- The breathing and silent mantra repetition is regulated into a 22-beat rhythm.

- Inhale in four equal parts (or sniffs) through the nose to make one full inhale, mentally repeating the mantra syllables 'Sa Ta Na Ma' with one syllable for each sniff.

- Hold your breath, mentally repeating 'Sa Ta Na Ma' four times for a total of 16 beats.

- Exhale all the breath through the nose for two beats while mentally repeating the mantra 'Wahe Guru'.

- Adjust the pace of the beats to be as slow as possible within your own comfortable breathing capacity but maintain the pace evenly across the 22-beat rhythm.

Classically, this practice is indicated for between 11 and 62 minutes, but effects may be seen with a shorter practice. If breath retention incites panic or difficulty, it is better to return to a practice without retentions at first.

RELAXATION-INDUCING ACUPRESSURE (MARMA)

From an Ayurvedic perspective, marmas are vital points in the body that may be manipulated to encourage balance and vibrant health (Frawley, Ranade and Lele, 2003). They correspond to terminus points of key nerves that send messages from the periphery of the body to the spinal cord and through to the brain. It is recommended that self-acupressure be done in a simple seated posture (sukhasana, as in the image below) or sitting in a chair with a straight back and feet firmly on the floor. These positions allow optimum flow of prana or energy. Here, we use two hand points and three points on the head, which I learnt from my colleague, Ayurvedic practitioner Jono Zondous.

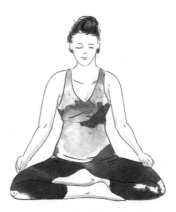

1. Two Marmas for Soothing and Grounding Heart Energy – Hand Points

These hand marma points are easy to do in bed and are subtle enough as an anti-anxiety/tension technique to use in public, from the office to a seat on public transportation. The effect of these marma points is a 'descending' or 'grounding' feeling. I've observed in my classes and sessions that when these are done properly around 90 per cent of the people who use them experience a profoundly relaxing and calming effect. This process can be repeated when you're getting off to sleep at bedtime or trying to get back to sleep having woken in the night. Remember to apply pressure to the marma on the inhale and release the pressure on the exhalation without creating tension or strain in the neck or shoulders.

These two hand points are said to have a profoundly releasing and relaxing effect on the internal organs, particularly on the uterus in women, and as such the hand points are not recommended during pregnancy.

Step by Step
CROOK OF THE HAND (KSHIPRA MARMA)

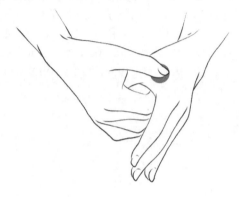

Kshipra marma or crook of the hand is found in the flesh between thumb and index finger.

- Apply pressure with the opposite thumb on inhaling and release the pressure on the exhale.

- You may wish to massage this point as you inhale, before releasing on the exhale.

- In general this point can be rather tender and, if you feel a response, you're in the right spot.

- This point quickly grounds the energy in the body, relieves mental tension and settles prana in the upper half of the body.

HEART OF THE HAND (TALA HRDAYA MARMA)

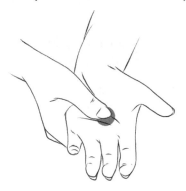

This location is known as the heart of the hand. According to Ayurveda, the mind has its seat in the heart and calls this *hrdayam*. In the Ayurvedic understanding, an imbalanced heart rhythm and energy often contribute to disturbed sleep.

- Feel around in the centre of your palm until you find the sensitive point.

- Again, apply pressure with your other thumb on the inhale and release the pressure on the exhale.

- Repeat for six cycles.

2. Three Marma Points to Get 'Out of Your Head'

Prana is said to be regulated by *sthapani* (awareness) of adhipati marma located at the third eye (ajna chakra) and crown of the head. These two marma points create a sense of focused relaxation. They also help to relieve tension in the face and dissipate eye strain.

Step by Step
FOCUS POINT

- Press **focus marma** above the top lip where the teeth meet the gums with your right index finger.

- Press the point on an inhalation, releasing the pressure on the exhalation. Repeat this six times.

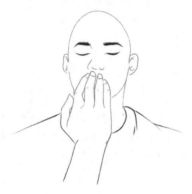

Focus Marma

THIRD EYE POINT

- Next move the index finger to the **third eye**, a little above and centred between the eyebrows.

- Feel for the notch.

- Press the point on the inhale, releasing on the exhale for six cycles.

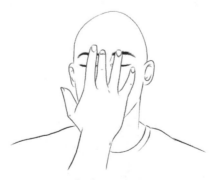

Third Eye Marma

CROWN CHAKRA POINT

- Take the palm of your right hand and place the little finger horizontal to the third eye measuring 12 finger breadths back to the top of the head.

- Locate the point corresponding to the **crown chakra**.

- Release here at this point by using three fingers to rub in an anti-clockwise circle steadily.

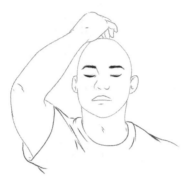

Crown of Head Marma

ACTIVATING/WAKE-UP BREATHING PRACTICES

These practices are presented in order – from the gentlest to the strongest. The first two of these practices, ujjayii with lengthened inhale and Surya Bhedana, can be done sitting down or even lying down on your back, and are variations on practices described in fuller detail above. The third – Breath of Joy – is a vigorous standing practice requiring a bit more space. For some of my clients and students, this is a firm morning wake-up favourite.

1. Soft Ujjayii with Lengthened Inhale

Following the instructions for the ujjayii breath as above, you may add a subtle stimulating and awakening aspect by lengthening the inhale slightly as compared with the exhale. It's best not to do this for too long as it can cause lightheadedness.

2. Surya Bhedana – Right Nostril Breathing
Step by Step

- Follow the instructions for Chandra Bhedana as described in the section on Alternate Nostril Breathing, above.

- For a stimulating effect, practise inhalation and exhalation through the right nostril, while gently blocking the left nostril.

- This may be done seated or lying down.

- Start with this breathing in and out for the same duration, or practise with a slightly lengthened inhalation uniformly throughout the practice for a gently stimulating effect.

3. Strong Invigorating Breath: Breath of Joy

This breath is very invigorating, energizing and stimulating. The movement of your arms and in-breath stretches the intercostal muscles in the ribcage, activating the rapid-acting stretch receptors in the lungs. According to Amy Weintraub (2004), a leading expert on yoga for depression, this breath has anti-depressive and mood-lifting qualities.

The first inhalation (arms forward) encourages diaphragmatic breathing. The second inhalation (arms to the side) encourages thoracic breathing, while the third inhalation (arms up) encourages clavicular breathing. While some may call the exhale 'detoxifying', I prefer to explain the exhale as releasing carbon dioxide, while the forward bend stretches the long muscles that line the spine.

I recommend doing the sequence with slightly bent knees, and bouncing on each part of the breath to add more vitality. I modify the out-breath forward bend by placing forearms or elbows inside the upper knee area to 'brace' the exhale, adding a slight brake to the forward bend instead of sending the arms through the centre of the legs. This helps to make the forward bend safer for anyone with back injuries, adds a grounding quality and minimizes lightheadedness.

Arms up (inhale), arms out (inhale), arms up (inhale).

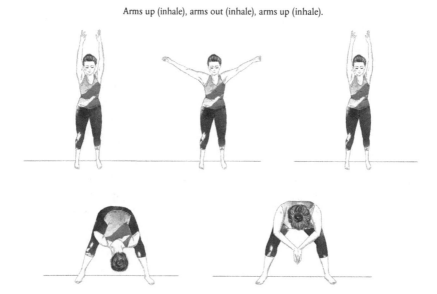

Forward bend (exhale) version 1 or forward bend (exhale) version 2.

Step by Step

- Stand with your feet wider than hip distance apart. Keep your knees bent gently or even bounce with the movements carried out below.

- Take three sharp 'sips' of breath in through your nose. Each 'sip' has a corresponding arm movement. You'll bend forward as you exhale. Use the more activating strong ujjayii breath for these.

- Sip 1. Inhale through the nose and gently swing your arms up in front of you, parallel to the floor.

- Sip 2. Inhale through the nose again, while swinging your arms open to the sides in a T shape, opening your chest.

- Sip 3. Inhale and lift your arms up with your hands overhead.

- Exhale. Exhale through your nose sharply while lowering your arms to rest on top of your thighs as you bend forward gently. Before the exhale you may choose to add a 'Ha' sound. This means you will exhale through your mouth.

The arm movements are: front, side, up, down. The breath movement is: in, in, in, out.

Contraindication notes: The Breath of Joy is not recommended for those with untreated high blood pressure, head injuries, migraines or glaucoma. For those with physical limitations, or who are easily over-stimulated by sympathetic nervous system activation, smaller movements can be made with the arms. For those with low blood pressure, it is important to keep a slower pace, and fold forward on the exhale more slowly.

Chapter Three

Mental Recovery

Mind *within* Matter

When people come to me with sleep problems, here are two of the most common things they say:

'I can't switch off my thoughts.'

and:

'I get into bed and my brain starts running a mile a minute.'

Before they begin the sleep recovery process, many of my insomniacs watch the clock tick the night away, trying desperately to clear their minds. If only they could 'switch off'. Anxious, fearful, repetitive, intrusive, stressful or just *plentiful* thoughts seem to come in a constant stream. Why, they ask, do I get this *parade* of thoughts before sleep or in the middle of the night? And what can I do about it?

It's essential that we *manage* and work *with* the mind, rather than try to switch it from 'on' to 'off'. One of the biggest lessons in this Sleep Recovery programme is that we can't treat ourselves like machines. This chapter looks at how to dissipate and deal with the mental activity that can prevent sleep, and how to recondition our mental patterns to help us to get to sleep and stay asleep more easily.

Doing this will address one of the biggest factors in insomnia: the fear factor. The *fear* of not sleeping well can shift a run of sleeplessness or interrupted sleep into full-blown insomnia. Our anxieties can start up – or lock in – a fear or stress response which then involves our neurochemistry and our physical state. Clearly the mind affects the body. In other words mind *affects* matter. Many of the common approaches to insomnia follow a 'mind-over-matter approach'. But the relationship is more interconnected. Our minds aren't the only aspects of ourselves influencing our bodies and our sleep. In fact we have seen how the body's position and tension affect the mind and emotions. Powerful sleep recovery results from working on the relationship between mind, body and all other aspects of ourselves.

Much like our bodies need to properly digest our food, we can view our minds as needing to assimilate and process all that they have ingested throughout the day. This chapter offers a method for doing just this. I call this 'mental digestion'. We'll also look at how *meditation* can help us get into the mental and physical states that help to initiate and support deep sleep. Instead of on/off, we might think of this as *downshifting* the brain from wakefulness into sleep through a state called the 'relaxation response'. We will explore two very simple methods that, when learnt and practised regularly, create powerful new patterns in consciousness.

While the traditional goal of yoga and meditation focuses on spiritual awakening, these practices help you to sleep by de-centring the daily concerns we encounter through the swipe and click of a smartphone, the ups and downs of getting and spending, and daily dramas. When we rest, we touch a part of ourselves far deeper and more elemental. In fact, the Sanskrit word for sleep, *svapna*, can be translated as 'close to the self'. When we learn to work with our minds compassionately, as part of the whole self, we learn valuable tools for better *svapna* – or closeness to the Self.

Improving 'Mental Digestion'

There is a common pattern in people who complain of sleep problems. One of my clients said this to me:

> All day long, I am inundated with information – I take in emails, calls, news sites, messaging apps, meetings. I'm seeing, hearing, speaking, formulating and responding quickly. My thoughts are always 'on'. Life is so fast I don't have time to take a break, and when I do, I find myself collapsing or numbing out. When I go on holiday, I find myself getting ill for the first part of it because I'm so exhausted. (Simon)

If we don't pause, it's like eating a great big meal without allowing any time to digest it. Food sits unprocessed in the stomach and gut, and the result is a very uncomfortable case of indigestion. Much of the unresolved or unprocessed mental material from the day comes back to revisit us when we slow our bodies down and become still, possibly for the first time all day. For most people this is when unprocessed or unresolved situations, thoughts or emotions crop back up. Several concepts and techniques in this chapter address the need to digest our thoughts and impressions from the day in order to put it all to bed at night.

No 'Off' Switch, But We Can Shift Our 'State of Mind'

The idea that we should be able to 'switch off' our minds is fundamentally flawed. People who get to sleep easily and stay asleep solidly appear to switch from 'on' to 'off' like machines. However, this is impossible. People who sleep easily are simply more adept at down-shifting smoothly and quickly from the waking state into a relaxed state, and then into deeper sleep states. There is no single magic button for powering down, though it is possible to manage – and decrease – the extent to which heightened mental activity prevents us from getting to sleep and interrupts sleep partway through the night. We may even be able to build our capacity to enter each needed rest state through practices that essentially re-train our brains. In this chapter we learn ways of managing these states of mental activity or 'consciousness' – working *with* the mind to first manage repetitive or anxious thoughts, and second, to repair the powering-down process.

This chapter outlines (1) major modern medical/psychological approaches, (2) yoga-based concepts of the mind as they relate to our sleep and (3) mind-based techniques for sleep recovery that draw upon the wisdom of both approaches in an embodied way. You'll learn simple, practical techniques that you can easily teach to your students or clients.

Traditional Mind-Over-Matter Cognitive Approaches

Traditional medical approaches to sleep have long focused on:

1. sleep hygiene to correct the habits that prevent good sleep

2. sleep rescheduling or sleep restriction

3. psycho-active medication.

Very good summaries of sleep restriction and rescheduling programmes are plentiful in the published literature, and these can be very helpful. In fact, without using the more strict and structural approaches, I have successfully implemented sleep restriction techniques with most of my clients – simply limiting time in bed to sleep-appropriate times and staying away from bed until sleepiness descends.

The holistic yoga therapy approach to sleep recovery in this book combines the first two components used in the medical model with a very different third element. We replace *pills* with *practices*, using yoga techniques that create neurochemical and physical changes that promote sleep immediately and in the longer term. Whereas sleeping pills become less effective over time, the yoga-based practices become more effective the more they are used. They create 'samskara' or 'grooves' – an idea that we will return to later in this chapter.

The mental habits and practices upon which we focus in this chapter, as well as the practices that recondition body, breath, nervous system and emotional response patterns towards sleep, are sustainable over the long term, and not only avoid harmful side effects, but also provide enduring benefits.

Cognitive Behavioural Therapy and CBT-I

Increasingly, psychological approaches have become more widely accepted in medical/health settings, as there is widespread acknowledgement that insomnia relates to mental activity. When applied to insomnia, CBT is referred to as CBT-I, adding the 'I' for insomnia. The over-riding principle of this approach to insomnia is 'mind over matter'.

While other psychological approaches are discussed in Chapter 4, we look at CBT here as it deals with thoughts and behaviours. It is popular as a treatment for insomnia for three reasons:

1. It is relatively short-term compared with traditional psychotherapy.

2. It is focused on issues and solutions.

3. It lends itself to greater standardization and adheres to the time and resource constraints of public health or private insurance systems.

According to the web site of the US-based non-profit, the National Sleep Foundation, CBT for insomnia involves behavioural changes (such as keeping a regular bedtime and wake-up time, getting out of bed after being awake for 20 minutes or so, and eliminating afternoon naps) and it adds a cognitive or 'thinking' component. CBT works to challenge unhealthy beliefs and fears around sleep and to teach rational, positive thinking.

Under the English National Health Service, CBT involves between 5 and 20 weekly or biweekly sessions lasting 30–60 minutes each in which client and therapist work to break down problems into their separate parts – thoughts, physical feelings and actions. Together, client and therapist seek to identify unrealistic or unhelpful patterns, determine how thoughts and habits interact, and work out how they affect the client. They develop a strategy for changing the unhelpful thoughts and behaviours. The client then takes home and puts into practice a plan of action, with follow-up in subsequent sessions. The emphasis is on applying the skills learnt during treatment. The goal is to manage problems and prevent them having a negative impact on life.

The US National Institute of Health's description of CBT-I also specifically includes the use of relaxation techniques and biofeedback to reduce anxiety, through better control of breathing, heart rate, muscles and mood. Biofeedback uses specific machines to gauge body functions, which some health insurance companies pay for, but which can be a drain on public health systems.

The CBT-based insomnia books and sleep techniques I've reviewed tend to be written by well-informed doctors and psychology professionals. Their treatment of self-initiated physical-or-breath-based relaxation techniques comprise *only about 1–2 per cent of the total text of their books*, effectively relegating these techniques to a side-note, for example two to three pages in a 250-page book. This may be due to the understandable unease with which medical professionals approach instructing clients or patients in physical movement. If this is true, it is logical – doctors are most often highly skilled in listening to complaints and then diagnosing and explaining conditions and prescriptions. However, cueing movement involves a different set of skills – one much more effectively developed if the instruction comes from a person who has experienced the movements, and has practised explaining them before. To effectively replace pills with practices,

I suggest an embodied, experiential approach – try the exercises, practise them and offer them.

From a yoga therapy perspective, it is also easy to see that rebalancing the over-active mind is far easier when the body is relaxed, feels safe, and there is good awareness of breathing. When we feel better physically, we have greater ease in changing our habits, as well. The structures of body and mind are far more rigid when we're under stress, and more malleable when we have come into a less-agitated state.

Retraining Your Brain: A Mind–Meditation–Sleep Theory

Building upon the knowledge that different brain wave patterns accompany different states of sleep, which we explored earlier, we turn to these patterns once again. The following is a set of theories that were developed in collaboration with Heather Mason of the Minded Institute. When we began collating client, course and workshop experience to crystallize into the Yoga Therapy for Insomnia continuing professional development (CPD) course, we began to look at the different brain wave patterns involved in sleep and compare them to what meditators experienced and practised in meditation, according to the existing research. Because of its documented impact on brain wave patterns, meditation may provide another important benefit for those with insomnia: it may facilitate the movement into brain wave patterns necessary to fall asleep and stay asleep.

A 'brain wave' is a name given to a particular type of activity in the brain that can be measured by a device called an electro-encephalogram (EEG). This device is placed on the scalp and picks up electrical activity in the brain as neurons send signals to each other. When we look at a section or all of the brain, this electrical activity appears wave-like. Faster electrical activity correlates with a particular type of wave and relates to particular brain functions and subjective experience. Similarly, slow waves correlate with other types of activity and experience.

Below are some examples of brain wave patterns that correspond to daily experiences.

Beta waves are associated with waking brain activity. Being able to tackle your to-do list and respond to emails efficiently but then being able to put it down during your break time shows balanced beta wave activity. Lying in the dark thinking about the previous day, and feeling anxiety or fear about past or upcoming events, may relate to over-active beta wave activity.

Alpha waves are associated with a relaxed waking state, or a transition from waking to sleeping. Sitting quietly, simply observing your breath or a pleasant view, listening to music without distraction or watching the kettle boil and feeling your feet on the floor might correspond with balanced alpha.

Theta waves are associated with the sleep state. When they are present in the waking state we may experience daydreaming, feeling little motivation and a desire to stare into space. Entering into a visionary state during meditation, visualization or a shamanic journey may represent an appropriate context involving high theta while awake.

Delta waves are the deepest sleep state, in which we dream. When feeling sluggish and brain-fogged in the morning, possibly due to an alarm going off in the middle of a dream, it may be that we are bringing a state of delta wave activity into the daytime.

Gamma waves are associated with experiences like watching a sunset and feeling touched by its beauty, seeing children at play and feeling their joy, appreciating the care of a friend or feeling happy for no reason.

Depending upon a person's disposition and their habits of body and mind, a person may tend towards being over-active or under-active in different brain wave states.

Not Switching Off But 'Dropping Down'

People who are highly stressed have a high concentration of beta waves and may struggle to drop into alpha as a precursor for cascading into the sleep states of delta and theta. Practising meditation may help individuals with insomnia start training the brain in the right ways to make the transition into sleep more easily – not switching off but 'dropping down'. Regular meditation practice helps us to reduce sympathetic nervous system activity and allow us to enter the relaxation-response state more easily.

Delta Waves, Dopamine and Sleep

There is another possible mechanism by which meditation may help to support sleep – the connection between dopamine and delta wave patterns. Those who experience insomnia, anxiety and depression have also been shown to have less of the neurotransmitter called dopamine, a 'feel good' neurotransmitter. Dopamine is released in anticipation of reward, during pleasurable experiences, and when people take narcotics like cocaine.

Drugs used to increase dopamine levels – such as those used for the treatment of Parkinson's disease – increase delta sleep. If we undertake activities that increase dopamine, we may also support better sleep through boosting delta activity. Activities that sustainably and healthily increase dopamine may help improve sleep, for example pleasant touch (self-massage or massage done by others), reward and praise.

Research also shows that a guided meditation technique called yoga nidra also increases dopamine levels. Yoga nidra practice may be useful in building dopamine, and therefore make delta sleep more accessible and deep over time. Clients may benefit from its incorporation in yoga therapy, and it can be an enjoyable and relaxing practice for those with the capacity to safely lie down with a recording or a teacher in a group setting. However, I do not make yoga nidra a part of this particular yoga therapy protocol because it relies on an external stimulus (a recording or teacher) to reap the benefits.

Yoga Perspectives on the Mind

The Western idea of the body–mind divide is relatively recent. The mind-over-matter techniques that arise from this way of thinking *can* offer valuable means of reducing anxieties and overwhelm that then lead to agitation in body, and prevent sleep. However, the dualistic model of 'I think, therefore I am' is limited and potentially unhelpful. If we see the mind as *embedded within the other 'layers' of ourselves*, we can utilize its connection to all of the self. Our range of tools expands, our ways of assisting the recovery process become more flexible, deep and sustainable.

The yoga tradition views the way we experience ourselves and the world as related to 'consciousness', generally speaking. It is fair to say that the yoga traditions were not explicitly concerned with therapeutic healing of health conditions but created techniques that guided the mind and perceptions away from daily concerns – either to still the mind completely or to reach transcendent states that were perhaps more aligned with divinity or unity. In fact, much of the meditation done by adepts in the spiritual traditions did not lead to sleep, but to awakening. At times, this awakening might have a fiery and active character, or an expansion into imaginal and spiritual realms with an airy nature, and only *sometimes* a deeply calming and peaceful tone. Meditation practices in spiritual lineages have many purposes, and our goal here is not to analyse them all, but to offer therapeutic approaches that help to heal the broken mechanisms of mind needed to enter a state of sleep.

As the yoga philosopher Georg Feuerstein (2011, p.83) notes, 'as soon as we try to quiet our minds, we tend to think of everything under the sun'. He continues:

> ...all the repressed and unassimilated psychic material of the day (and of long ago) bubbles up forcing our consciousness to seek relief by externalizing through the senses... We can greatly reduce the mind's tendency to externalize attention by cultivating a balanced, calm disposition at all, times not merely for a few minutes a day.

The yogic principle of 'detachment' is possible when we don't *believe* all the mind's stories but develop a relationship to the thinking mind that goes beyond each individual thought.

Mental Constitution and Sleep, According to Ayurveda

In Ayurvedic thinking (Lad, 2007), the mind becomes imbalanced due to inappropriate diet, inappropriate lifestyle, lack of clarity in relationships, repressed emotions and stress (excessive responsibility, boredom, etc.). There are three constitutions of mind according to this perspective:

- Sattva – peaceful and balanced. Sleep in a person with a sattvic mind is sound but alert.

- Rajas – fiery and active. A rajasic person's sleep is light and is often interrupted or disturbed by dreams.

- Tamas – slow and steady. A tamasic person sleeps for long periods of deep sleep and loves daytime naps.

Our yoga forebears were able to glean from observation a phenomenon that modern science has demonstrated through data from EEG and observation of brain waves. We have several states, which the yoga traditions related to different aspects of mind. According to yogic understanding, in the waking state the part of the 'mind' called Manas is active – in this state we gather impressions through the outer thinking and perceiving faculties (Manas) and the senses. In the dream state, we digest impressions through our inner intelligence (Buddhi), and these are reflected through our subtle senses in the form of dreams. Dreams are said to show the process of mental digestion. In the deep sleep state the residue of our digested impressions, reduced to seed form, becomes part of our deeper consciousness (Chitta) (Frawley, 2005). The yogic understanding also suggests that a transcendental state, which pervades all the other mental states, can lead to awakening or enlightenment. Through yoga we can move beyond a stressed-out and preoccupied mind, to find new states of mind and broader awareness.

The Mind in the Yoga Sutras

One of the early stanzas in the Yoga Sutras, 'Yogas chitta vrtti nirodha', is often translated as 'yoga is the stilling of the fluctuations of the mind'. The translation may lead modern yoga practitioners to the misleading conclusion that it is possible to stop thinking as easily as turning off a switch, with a few postures and breathing practices. The classical and traditional definitions of yoga were philosophical and spiritual in nature, with practices designed to pull attention away from the outward senses and 'turn inward' for purposes as diverse as seeing and experiencing beyond the material plane, engaging in alchemical transformation or identifying with the universal or divine. In a sense, entering the mind-state that allows us to sleep is a way of letting go of the logical-thinking mind and allowing a more spacious aspect of the mind to take over.

As discussed in the previous chapters, both asana and pranayama do have profound effects on the mind. The mental faculties of both concentration and knowledge are required in order to perform the practices. The more subtle movements of the mind are referred to in the limbs of yoga called pratyahara and dharana. Pratyahara refers to moving our senses from external objects to the inward awareness. Dharana may be translated as 'container' or a place to put the mind.

TOOLS FOR MANAGING THE MIND
About the Practices

Self-guided practices described in this chapter act to balance and prepare the mind for sleep. They help build the capacity to shift mental states from waking through to deep sleep. One great tool is meditation. The other is writing.

Mindfulness and meditation develop a relationship to our senses, so that we are not simply flooded by them. Coming into present-time awareness can dissipate our stress responses. We use simple focusing meditation practices that, when practised regularly, increase our capacity to enter states of calm, relaxed awareness and reinforce our ability to move from the waking state into deep sleep with ease. One practice here focuses on the breath as the 'dharana' or container for awareness, while the other uses mantra, an internally repeated syllable, as its 'vehicle'.

Writing can be used to start the process of slowing down the mind, and seeing what it contains. This can help us to right-size and adjust perceptions that are unhelpful and can seem all-consuming. Many of my clients find that if they write down their ruminations, jotting down the thoughts they find turning over in their minds before bed, this helps them get to sleep more easily and effectively.

WRITING

Cathy, who is retired and has suffered from sleep problems for many years, says, 'I was always exhausted and couldn't seem to think straight all day, but when I'd get into bed at night, my mind would become a three-ring circus of every possible thought imaginable: family birthdays, managing my daily diary so that I have enough but not too much to do, replaying conversations with my kids.' Cathy began to do some journalling before her bedtime yoga routine and found that her mind was more settled and it was easier to focus on her breathing as she moved. With a more settled mind, the stretches seemed to go deeper. If during her morning wake-up routine, particularly focused on anti-depressive postures and breath, she had intrusive thoughts or felt preoccupied, she'd write down the daily to-dos and found that not only was her sleep improving because the morning practices brought stimulation at the right time of day, but she was finding it easier to manage enjoyable daily activities, be more creative with her (many) grandchildren's birthday gifts, feel less preoccupied and more 'on top of things'.

MEDITATION

Simon notices that, when he wakes up in the middle of the night, all manner of things come to him. He might fixate upon a situation at work, where, as managing director, he feels the full weight of responsibility. Many a strategy and plan has been hatched while the world sleeps. While it's great to have some peace and quiet to get his thoughts in order, he wishes it didn't have to come at the expense of his sleep. With Simon's fiery personality, he is capable of personal discipline when he is provided with a credible and demonstrable benefit, rationale and plausible plan. Many years of research evidence on Transcendental Meditation plus my own explanation of how it's helped me in my own sleep recovery are enough for Simon to say he will give it a go. He is not the type to say yes to something he won't do, and when he says he's going to do something, he does it.

We look together at his daily schedule, and identify two periods in which he can do a 20-minute meditation. The first is after his morning drive into work. He can park his car at the park near his office, and in good weather meditate on a bench. On gloomy or rainy days, he gets out of the driver's seat and sits on the passenger side, locks the doors and closes his eyes there. After work he has made a plan with his wife and children that he will say hello, go directly up to his room for 20 minutes, meditate and then come back down to greet the family and begin his evening. During this time, he 'burns through' many thoughts and the events of the day, usually in the first 10–15 minutes of his meditation. Over time, he's noticed that his system seems to settle for at least a few minutes and he is able to find a state of rest and calm, and often has a creative thought or memory bubble to the surface. Simon finds that these buffers at the start and end of his workday leave him refreshed, focused and more present – first for meeting the challenges of a demanding job, and then allowing the workday to be dispatched so that it doesn't bleed into family time, and he's more present for his wife and kids. He's noticed that, at bedtime, he's more relaxed and less likely to encounter the 'parade of thoughts', and wakes in the middle of the night for 'problem solving' far less frequently, and usually only when he has a glass of wine with dinner.

1. Journalling Guidelines

Many of my clients and students experience the bedtime 'thought parade'. When it's time to put our bodies into the bed at the end of a long, busy day, it can be the only time we've stopped and had a chance to process the day at all. Any thoughts, worries, resentments, concerns or slights can arise very naturally and cause anxiety, worry or simple preoccupation. They've been waiting all day for attention.

I suggest that clients keep a journal in which they can do a brain-dump, reviewing the day, and setting aside anything that needs to be noted for tomorrow – without getting into an exhaustive to-do list. If something inter-personal is causing concern, write it down. If something at work is unsettled, write it down. Write thoughts, intuitions and the sense of the situation, and keep writing until you are ready to set it aside. For some people, they need to feel that no one will find their brain-dump, in which case I suggest tearing it up, or disposing of it before bed or in the morning. Others find keeping a journal to which they can refer later very helpful for resolving the difference between late-night anxieties – which are often disproportionate – and daytime reality.

2. External Awareness Mindfulness: The BELL Technique

The BELL technique, from my colleague Dr Barbara Mariposa (2018), author of the *Mindfulness Playbook*, stands for Breathe, Expand your awareness, Listen, Look. This simple practice takes your mind out of story-mode and brings you into your senses in the present moment. It's very, very simple. You don't even need to close your eyes. You can do this practically any time, provided you're in a generally safe environment. Even if there's something emotional happening, you can practise this and start to shift your brain chemistry.

Step by Step

- Breathe simply and easily.

- Take two or three deep breaths and then expand your awareness.

- Become aware of what is happening around you – even notice what's happening to your body, notice what's happening in the room.

- Maybe you can even look out a window and see what is there.

- When you look, notice three things that you can see, perhaps an object, or a colour. Doing this brings you into the pre-frontal cortex of the brain.

- Then see what three things you can hear when you listen. These are things that bring you into the present moment, take you out of stress and bring you into a more rested state.

- You may continue the exercise to note three things you can touch, smell or even taste.

- Keep it simple and practise it often to come back to present-time mindfulness.

3. Meditation to Enter the Relaxation Response

Meditation can be very simple. This does not mean that in practice it is easy! The basics of meditation involve very little. Gently guiding the wandering mind back to a chosen focus is one of the main keys to the meditation process. That action of the mind seems to train the brain to have thoughts and not allow them to cause distress, but to come back to centre and enter a relaxed state. This can prove very helpful when the mind experiences a stream of thoughts at sleep time. Sat Bir Khalsa, in his mini-book *Your Brain on Yoga* (Khalso with Gould, 2012), summarizes how to meditate to enter the Relaxation Response in two simple steps.

Step by Step

- Select a word, mantra or your breath, etc. and focus your attention on it in a relaxed manner.

- When other, everyday thoughts intrude (and they will), let them go and bring your attention once again to the first step in a relaxed and patient manner, letting go without frustration or judgement.

4. Simple Breath Meditation Technique – Internal Awareness

This form of meditation centres on 'mindfulness of breathing'. It is a form of Buddhist meditation now common to Tibetan, Zen, Tiantai and Theravada Buddhism as well as Western-based mindfulness programmes. 'Ānāpānasati' means *to feel the sensations caused by the movements of the breath in the body* as is practised in the context of mindfulness. According to tradition, Ānāpānasati was originally taught by Gautama Buddha. The technique here is not essentially different from the two steps noted above; the process is simply fleshed out a bit more here, focusing on the breath, while the meditation technique that follows focuses on a mantra.

Benefit

This is particularly useful as a form of meditation for those who have difficulty with overwhelming thoughts that disturb the first phase of sleep. The simple, single point in the body – essentially at the third eye point – helps to slow down the mind, creating a more spacious awareness. It has the ability to begin calming the system effectively and quickly.

Step by Step

- Sit quietly and comfortably, unmoving but not forcing yourself to sit so still that you feel tense.

- Bring your attention to the breath as it enters the nostrils, particularly inside the nose, where there is a bit of moisture in the mucous membrane.

- Begin by noticing the temperature, texture, moisture and quality of the air moving in and out of your nose.

- Stay with this awareness, and when your mind goes elsewhere, gently bring it back to the inside of the nose.

- Observe the breath without altering the inhalation or exhalation, noticing the 'arising and passing' of the breath as well as of the thoughts.

- Stay here for between 10 and 20 minutes and do this as a regular practice.

5. Mantra Meditation Technique

This form of meditation is widespread and long established in the West. The technique involves the use of a simple syllable or phrase repeated inwardly, over and over in the mind, without grasping on or forcing the mind to repeat it. It is based on manas (mind) + tra (as in the word 'traverse', meaning 'to move across'). Mantra is seen as a vehicle that holds or carries the mind. The mantra is held lightly and the mind directed back to the mantra when thoughts arise.

This technique, like the meditation technique above, has a wide range of benefits, including:

- greater inner calm throughout the day

- reduced cortisol (the 'stress hormone')

- normalized blood pressure

- reduced insomnia

- lower risk of heart attack and stroke

- reduced anxiety and depression

- improved brain function and memory.

Finding, Choosing or Being Given a Mantra

Most long-established meditation lineages involve a teacher giving a mantra to the student. It is highly recommended that an experienced and seasoned meditation teacher offers the practices to a student for many reasons. One is said to centre on the understanding of the 'vibrational' effects of a mantra, much like a medicine being prescribed to a patient. If we consider the Ayurvedic notion that we have different constitution types and qualities of mind, as discussed in this book, it makes sense that a mantra will not be one-size-fits-all, or one for every constitution of body or mind.

Another reason for a mantra being passed down from teacher to student may have to do with the importance of the student learning from the *embodied state of the meditation teacher*. Meditative state is seen as being conveyed to the student through what the yogis called 'transmission'. This may have something to do with spiritual conveyance or may be explained through our modern understanding of *mirror neurons*, which enable us to pick up on the states of others through neurophysiological means.

The Transcendental Meditation or Vedic Meditation method involves receiving a mantra from the teacher, and once initiated into its use, the meditator uses this same mantra to meditate for 20 minutes twice daily. The first practice is done in the morning before activity has begun, and the second in the afternoon before the evening meal. The commitment and focus that meditation brings helps to regulate sleep by having profound effects at two essential times of the day: upon waking and in the mid-afternoon slump. The benefits can be understood in terms of both 'purification', in allowing thoughts to arise and be processed and cleared out, and in terms of 'deep rest', which may occur when the meditator feels like she is falling asleep.

Step by Step

- Sit comfortably for a short period of time.

- Begin with the intention to think a simple syllable (the mantra).

- Bring the mantra into the mind; when the mind wanders, bring the mantra back.

- Do this without setting a timer. If you are curious about how much time has passed, look at your watch or clock. Doing this eventually develops the internal time-sense which may be helpful for sleep and wake disorders.

- After 20 minutes have passed, take a 2–3-minute 'buffer' without the mantra, in order to return to regular waking consciousness.

Chapter Four

Emotional Recovery for Sleep

Many of my clients have come to discuss insomnia but are in fact in some form of emotional distress: they are anxious, angry, sad or tense about life decisions or events, or are conflicted between head and heart. This may be a form of disturbed sleep that they consider 'insomnia' but it is really a very human and entirely natural response to strong emotions and upset. It is vital that we consider the emotional layer or 'the wisdom body' (which I equate in our five-layered system with the fourth layer, the vijnanamaya kosha). This chapter has two parts. In **Part A** we explore the ways in which our emotions can cause sleepless nights. I offer you tools to manage and work through the emotional causes of sleep disturbances. In **Part B** we look at trauma and post-traumatic insomnia, which are emotional, mental and physical in their nature. You'll find guidelines for working with insomnia when it is part of a trauma response – both in for one to one work and in teaching group yoga classes.

Part A: Emotions Can Cause Sleepless Nights
Life Transitions

Some life events inherently disrupt sleep because they interrupt our schedules and life rhythms: the birth or adoption of a child, travelling frequently for work or pleasure, a move to a new climate, or sharing a bed with a new partner, to name a few. Some transitions may involve emotional pain as well as changing logistics, which can amplify the impact of difficult times on our sleep. These include relationship breakups, the loss of a job or occupation, retirement, or children leaving the home. At times like these, painful memories may link to similar past events and long-stored emotions may be stirred up, upsetting our emotional balance.

Blocking Emotion Creates Stress

Many of my clients who come for yoga therapy have learnt that it isn't safe or 'good' to feel negative emotions. The psychologist Carl Rogers (1961), the father of person-centred psychotherapy, discussed how we learn to be 'incongruent': not matching our external actions and expression to what we feel on the inside. This can begin in childhood when parents respond to crying children by telling them 'don't cry' or 'don't be sad'. Perhaps they feel they have somehow failed if their little one is unhappy – perhaps we all feel discomfort when witnessing negative emotions. This occurs in many life circumstances. Indeed, 'professionalism' and/or 'good manners' may dictate that we hide or deny sadness, fear or anger in work or social settings. Some people learnt that particular emotions were unpalatable to their parents or families. This can have the effect of disconnecting us from our body-sense and our emotions from what we express on the outside. We may even go so far as to shut off conscious awareness of emotions if they are not acceptable to us, or to others.

Those who practise yoga postures or meditation, depending upon how they have been taught, may expect that yoga practice will remove negative feelings such as anger, rage, fear, grief, resentment and regret. Some may believe that the 'spiritual' aspects of yoga suggest that we do not feel negative emotions or seek to avoid feeling them. When emotions are avoided, deeper fears and anxieties and their causes may go unaddressed. Addressing our emotional needs more directly can lead to a decrease in unconscious tension that can cause sleeplessness directly, or result in activities used to distract oneself from the difficult emotions that arise during the quiet time before sleep or in the middle of the night.

To address the emotional aspects of sleeplessness, I offer three things:

1. a personal practice that links body sensation to emotion

2. a suggested communication strategy that many of my students and clients find transforms their personal relationships for the better

3. a prompt to refer onward for counselling or psychotherapy if emotional issues are at the heart of sleep problems.

What's important here is that there are aspects of ourselves that exist more deeply than our conscious thoughts which cognitive behavioural and purely physical approaches may not address.

Personality, Emotional Reaction and Sleep

Emotions can affect out sleep in different ways. Even if a person does not identify as having insomnia or sleeping problems, most people who are experiencing anger, sadness or other difficult emotional states will see some changes in their sleep. Some people deal with stress and upset by needing more sleep than usual, or by a sense of exhaustion that makes them take to their beds, never quite feeling refreshed for the greater duration of sleep. Other people find that it's more difficult than usual to drop off to sleep, while there are some who wake in the middle of the night after just a few hours and are unable to get back to sleep as they feel too agitated or upset. When emotionally driven changes to our sleep patterns become entrenched because they cause us to fear sleep, to worry about it or to establish 'secondary' habits that sabotage sleep, insomnia that meets a diagnostic level can result.

Some people experience emotions intensely and may be more aware that they are upset, making the link between their state and their sleeplessness. Others may be unaware of unprocessed emotional issues, which can drive physical or mental difficulties, including insomnia. Unexpressed emotions can be trapped in the body as tension and somatized into illnesses, or they can cause acting out in terms of negative reactions in relationship to others, addictions or other self-sabotaging behaviours, all of which can undermine sleep.

Returning to the constitutional types discussed in the Introduction, Vasant Lad (2007, p.166) explains the differences in the emotional tendencies of each of the three main types from an Ayurvedic perspective. While each person will experience a full range of emotions in their lifetime, in this view, the different constitutional types tend towards some emotions more than others. It can be useful to understand these tendencies, as a yoga therapeutic approach to better sleep, from the standpoint of emotions, would be to allow in those shadow emotions that are not able to be felt and expressed constructively, finding appropriate tolerance for their presence and constructive outlets into which the emotion may be channelled.

- A person with a predominantly airy, **vata** constitution tends towards emotions such as fear, insecurity and anxiety. A vata's emotions may seem unpredictable. One moment the person will cry, the next they will laugh. A vata person is more likely to find it hard to let go due to fear.

- A **pitta** person's fiery emotional state normally tends towards aggression, irritability, judgement and anger when out of balance. A pitta person will feel attachment but will move on quickly when it is time to say goodbye.

- A **kapha** person is often calm, but feels greed, possessiveness and attachment due to their earthy nature. It is very difficult for a kapha person to say goodbye because they feel sadness due to their attachment.

An individual's personality and character will often underpin the way in which they experience and react to life events and transitions.

> **Paul** was in his late fifties, and a successful investment banker. He is an avid runner, has two school-aged children, and recently went through an acrimonious divorce. Paul was always on the go, 'burning the candle at both ends', with many characteristics of the pitta personality and body type. Most nights Paul had trouble falling asleep and would wake after three hours in bed, inflamed with anger, turning over in his mind the conflict between himself and his ex-wife and their arguments about the children. He felt ragged, argumentative and desperate for sleep. His work intensity did not let up, and soon Paul found himself lashing out at a colleague before an important meeting, leading to a trip to the HR department and conversations about his health and wellbeing.
>
> Paul's doctor prescribed him some sleeping tablets and told him to take action to lower his stress levels. He began working with a mindfulness app on his phone, which he used twice daily, but still was unable to sleep well, and the anger didn't shift.
>
> He came for one-to-one yoga therapy for insomnia sessions. He didn't want to talk about the social aspects of his life, but knew that the insomnia was making him testy. I taught him the Simple Sleep Sequence, and three-part breathing. He began regular meditation. The change was dramatic – he appeared much calmer and tapered off sleeping tablets

medication with the help of his doctor. His ability to get to sleep improved, but he still woke in the middle of the night frequently, at times with his heart pounding, and other times sweating, both of which distressed him.

The yoga practices slowed Paul's nervous system down, and allowed him to build the capacity to allow in and sit with uncomfortable emotions. I asked him to track his state and he reported back feeling alternately impatient, tearful and angry in meditation. He asked if this was the sort of thing to discuss with a therapist. I told him this was exactly the thing to discuss with a therapist and found him a referral close to his home.

Paul began to talk with a therapist about his divorce, about loss, and his fears about being separated from his children and about being alone. He took responsibility for his part in his marriage breakdown and found a way to reframe his understanding of his ex-wife's part in the divorce. Paul began to see that his personal life had been on warp speed – running away from pain and assigning blame to himself and others. In therapy, Paul realized that he hadn't slept well for long stretches when, as a child, his parents left his native Germany for his father's new job in London, leaving him frightened, alone and resentful. Paul worked through the pain of separation as an adult, which mirrored losing contact with his friends and grandparents as a child.

As Paul began to explore the roots of his fears and anger, he began to use the 'emotional release meditation' I taught him in between therapy sessions. This helped him to alleviate the pressure created by the intensity of his life transition. He would use this technique alongside the yoga practices, particularly when he had to be in contact with his ex-wife and children. This has helped him to relax, his sleep has improved dramatically and he rarely wakes up in the middle of the night. Paul knows that if he feels tension in his body while trying to get to sleep or if he wakes upset, he can use the tools he's learnt in our work together, and no longer adds to his distress by worrying about insomnia. His panic attacks have not resurfaced, and he is feeling greater sadness at times, but also more happiness. He says he feels he's 'more real' and 'down to earth' in what he expects from himself and his life.

Emotions, Expansion and Contraction: The Concept of Spanda

How do emotions affect our bodies? One key way is through the mechanisms of contraction and expansion. This goes back to Sigmund Freud's early thinking: when we have an emotion or a thought, our bodies respond by expanding (opening up, relaxing and settling) or contracting (tightening, tensing and feeling more guarded or agitated). Aversion to something causes us to shrink away from it. Fear causes us to protect ourselves by tensing up. Similarly, if we have learnt that sadness, grief, regret, anger and other emotions are to be feared or are not acceptable, we will similarly tighten or tense against those emotions. When we feel enjoyable or positive emotions, for example when we receive a hug from someone we love, are praised, celebrate a success or feel accepted, we tend towards physical opening and expansion. If the overall emotional balance is tightening us, we feel less relaxed, less safe and less able to sleep. Our nervous systems respond by tipping into either hyper-arousal or shut-down.

The yoga traditions relate this to the nature of all creation. Human beings, like all things in nature, experience expansion and contraction. This natural pulsation, which is embodied in heartbeat and breath, is termed 'Spanda'. While tension and relaxation happen naturally, when the balance in our bodies tips into tension without enough relaxation, naturally our sleep is inhibited.

There is an old adage: 'What you resist will persist.' This is the case with difficult emotions. Negative emotions give rise to tension, and when that tension is not dissipated, it can lead to the hyper-arousal that can cause us to lose sleep. Both trouble falling asleep and waking in the middle of the night may be caused by this type of distress. Emotions can be far less conscious than thoughts, and we may push aside nascent feelings such as sadness, anger, fear, grief and resentment during the rush of daily life because they don't make sense and are inherently irrational or unacceptable to us. In fact, when we are asleep, our logical-rational functions diminish, making emotional upset both more prevalent and harder to dismiss.

A 2010 TED Talk by Brene Brown on the topic of vulnerability has over 32 million views. It has clearly hit a nerve for many people. In this talk Brown describes how, when we try to push away fears, anger, sadness, grief and mourning, all the negative parts of the spectrum of emotion, we start to numb ourselves. She describes how we shut down our capacity to feel, tightening ourselves up against the scary emotions. According to Brown, in order to be able to experience the positive states such as joy, love and wonder – which relate to feeling expansive and safe, relaxed and at ease – we have to develop tools to experience the negative end of the spectrum as well. As she states, 'We cannot selectively numb ourselves to emotion' if we are to be healthy.

While it is healthy to make unconscious negative emotions more conscious, it is also healthy to keep positive states in the forefront of our mind. Practices that involve recalling the things that are positive, for example creating 'gratitude lists' or practices of appreciation for what one has, can shift one's neurochemistry into a more favourable state for releasing tension and experiencing the expansive and relaxed states needed for sleep. When we feel happier, we tend to be more relaxed and sleep more easily.

We can assist our clients in sleeping more easily and soundly by recognizing the emotional roots of tension, offering simple strategies as outlined in this chapter, or by offering referrals to formally psychologically trained counsellors or therapists to help them to manage emotional difficulty. Psychological approaches tend to favour expression and resolution of challenging emotions, often by addressing reactions in response to expectations or events that occurred long in the past. Whether or not you are a psychologist, therapist or counsellor, your client may raise issues of concern such as marriage/relationship difficulties, work anxieties, family troubles, social isolation or overwhelm. You may also see a repeating pattern in their response to difficulties in that they may tend towards sadness/ despondency, towards an anger response, or towards anxiety. In these cases it may be useful to reflect back that this is an area with which a counsellor or psychotherapist may provide useful assistance in working through the issue or their response. People who have not considered therapy before may find it useful if repeated concerns are mirrored back to them gently, and if they are made aware that these are the sorts of concerns that counselling and therapy can assist them with. In some cultures and communities there may be a misperception that therapy is only for those who are severely mentally ill, perhaps confusing psychotherapy with the branch of medicine called psychiatry, or they may have the misperception that therapy is only for people who feel or act 'crazy'. Clearing up this confusion and de-stigmatizing counselling and therapy, and encouraging them to find a qualified professional with whom to work, may help your clients to resolve the sleep issues that emerge from ongoing difficulties with emotional processing.

In addition to referring onward where appropriate, we can offer yoga practices that balance the emotional tendencies that we see in our clients. Drawing upon the sister science of yoga, Ayurveda, we may see our clients as going 'out of emotional balance' more easily in one or more ways. For example, those who deal with negative life circumstances by responding with anger are very different from those who respond with a depressive state or by becoming anxious.

Towards Emotional Balance: The Yamas and Niyamas of Yoga

If better emotional balance leads to better sleep, then living a life that minimizes discord, includes self-awareness and features personal responsibility for creating harmony seems a good idea. In many contemporary yoga trainings, one of the most cited teachings on yoga's application to daily life is in Patanjali's Yoga Sutras – the yamas and niyamas. In the 'limbs' of yoga, the attitudinal orientations to daily life precede the physical, breath and meditative practices. In any spiritual practice, there are guidelines on behaviour as an expression of spiritual values in action. A classical interpretation of the Yoga Sutras relates to a spiritual practice of purification through renouncing worldly endeavours. However, this is not the purpose of yoga therapy. We instead look to the Yoga Sutras and adapt the tenets to living day-to-day lives involving work, family, relationships and other 'householder' engagements. However, in both contexts, the yamas and niyamas can provide a useful starting point for keeping our internal and external worlds in alignment. When we are in good alignment, this tends to give rise to a clear conscience and to minimize the negative impact of the difficulties and joys that life inevitably presents. Put another way: when we are out of alignment with our ethics or values or have become imbalanced in our habits, this can lead to sleep-sabotaging distress. While this is not an exhaustive checklist that I use with most clients, I keep these tenets in the back of my mind for noticing areas in which a client may be imbalanced. For those who tend to sleep well normally, a crisis of integrity, an inter-personal conflict or difficult work situation can cause one or more sleepless nights, or even a period of insomnia. If not carefully dealt with, the emotional genesis of a sleep problem may persist, or may lead to the habits that further entrench sleep problems.

Yamas

These may be interpreted as ways in which we treat all entities – including other people, ourselves, beings, animals and objects. When we relate as harmoniously as possible with others and with ourselves, we can rest with a clear conscience.

Ahimsa (non-harming): Acting in violent or harmful ways towards others or towards oneself creates conflict and often begets further violence. Doing harm to others can result in an unclear conscience or lead to further conflict. For many people who have difficulty sleeping, non-harming relates to something more subtle: the internalized critical voices that cause a person to view themselves harshly or to 'beat oneself up' can lead to perpetual tension, making it hard to rest. When the mind is at war with the heart, or a person feels like nothing they do is good enough for themselves or others, this is a form of emotional self-harming. In terms of sleep, ahimsa, when interpreted in the physical sense, may be interpreted as 'not contradicting the flow of nature' or maintaining habits that run counter to our circadian rhythms – as going against our biological programming for sleep is a way in which we may do harm to ourselves.

Satya (truthfulness): We tend to sleep better at night when we are genuine and authentic. Acting with integrity and honesty, not lying, not concealing the truth and not downplaying or exaggerating can maintain a clear conscience. This may take the form of being truthful with ourselves about our own needs. For example, admitting to oneself when we are actually tired, instead of staying up too late, is a form of truthfulness.

Asteya (non-stealing): Conflict is caused when we take what doesn't belong to us – money, goods, or credit for someone's work or status. If we steal others' property or engage in illegal actions, the threat of punishment may loom, causing fear or paranoia, two enemies of sleep. On a physical and more subtle level, in the previous chapters we explored 'borrowing from the energy credit card', which is a way of thinking about stimulants to gain energy through unsustainable means, depleting our stores, and robbing our reserves.

Brahmacharya (sexual restraint, or ethical conduct): Traditional sources equate brahmacharya with celibacy. The Yoga Sutras primarily dealt with those seeking yoga for enlightenment; in a rarefied environment like an ashram devoted to spirituality, this is a traditional practice. However, for those in householder daily life, this may be interpreted as restraint in sexual dealings, behaving responsibly and non-addictively with respect to sexual energy. Several of my clients report 'using' sexual release through intercourse or masturbation as a way to relax enough to get to sleep. This is not inherently problematic unless it is distorted, or the person becomes dependent upon it, if it causes addictive use of sexual energy or objectifies one's partner. Getting into ethical messes due to sexual impropriety can surely cause one to lose sleep! On a more subtle level, this can also relate to eros as creative energy – and mis-spending this creative energy can lead to feeling blocked or depleted.

Aparigraha (non-clinging): This tenet relates to not letting go. Being able to let go of possessions, status and other circumstances is helpful. An inability to let go of objects, people and circumstances can create tremendous difficulty, as no life situation is ever permanent. This can be a difficult practice and relates to not coveting what one doesn't have, and also not depending too heavily on what one does have. Related to sleep, holding on or greed may show up as a need to be in control. We may cling to being awake as a form of control because we don't feel safe in release. In order to receive sleep and rest, we need to loosen our grip on life, and learn to 'let go'. This doesn't come from repeating words, but from embodying the release of tension and working-through of emotional difficulties.

Niyamas or Internal Observances

Classically, these are seen both as practices and states of being that lead to 'samadhi' or enlightenment. Here they are reinterpreted to relate to our sleep.

Saucha (purity): Cleanliness of the internal state and our external environment begets good sleep. A diet free from excessive stimulants, toxic chemicals and junk, as well as a clutter-free, wholesome environment and cleanliness in one's business and personal dealings, can promote personal balance and healthy sleep.

Santosha (contentment): Equanimity, peace, tranquillity and accept-ance may not be our everyday state – but they can become practices that lead to these qualities becoming more accessible. When we focus on acceptance of our life circumstances and adapt to pain or loss by returning to a state of contentment where possible, it is easier to live a life conducive to repose and rest.

Tapas (passionate pursuit of spiritual awakening): Traditionally, tapas is seen as the 'heat of transformation' or passion related to spiritual practice. It can be related to the quality of discipline. Without tapas and desire for change, we may not break out of a rut, and the stagnancy of staying in an unhealthy situation can lead to insomnia. Those who exercise regularly and expend appropriate effort may sleep more easily than those who are sedentary or undisciplined. However, effort must be in balance with the other qualities like santosha (contentment) lest we overdo our efforts and burn out!

Svadhyaya (study of the self): Self-inquiry, mindfulness, self-study and the study of the yogic texts were part of the traditions of yoga. Self-awareness and study can lead to greater insight and clarity. Learning from the healing and introspective traditions can lead us to see sleeplessness as a symptom of some aspect of soul or spirit that is seeking balance or expression. Self-study can mean the difference between *suffering* from insomnia and seeing the bigger perspective, utilizing it as a wake-up call and taking action to look at one's wellbeing and life.

Ishvara Pranidhana (surrender to the Lord/universe/divine/nature): This tenet relates to our sense of context – that there is something greater than our individual control and agency: a self in relationship to God, nature or the universe. Letting go and surrender are at the heart of good sleep, in which we respond to our natural rhythms, and we can trust in the 'universe' or nature enough to release into sleep.

As we have seen, emotions run even deeper than conscious thought and the mind: they connect to the heart. We may think one thing but feel something else entirely. How authentic, 'congruent' and well aligned we are during the day can have a bearing on how we sleep at night. In the yoga tradition, there are many tools and techniques for everything from 'transcending negativity' to 'sitting with' negative emotions and allowing them to transform. I offer a gentle guide to some yoga therapy approaches that help to bring emotional balance.

Emotional Digestion and Processing

For those with trouble sleeping, constant movement through our life, busyness with work or family responsibilities can leave us reeling with problems, solutions and interpretations. Until it comes time to lie down in bed, many people are not aware of their emotions. Unless there is a readily available practice of going into stillness and quiet, we don't always give scope and space to emotions. Often, the only time we may give ourselves to be quiet is in the moments before sleep. What happens? Undigested emotional material, in the form of thoughts, can come flooding back in before bed, or can form the content of anxious or nervous feelings if we are awakened in the middle of the night.

Sitting with and Moving through Emotion

There are neurophysiological bases of anxiety and depression and certain neurotransmitter deficiencies (serotonin, dopamine, GABA) are involved. In addition, cortisol and adrenaline build up in the system and can lead to a state of anger, or be expressed as rage. However, we must look deeper to the emotional aspect of these insomnia-precipitating and insomnia-caused conditions. When we take the opportunity to allow these emotional states to arise, to be witnessed, received and moved through with awareness, our capacity to let go changes our sleep fundamentally. A calm comes to the system when we stop bracing ourselves against feeling and allow emotions to be felt. The Buddhist tradition of Vipassana refers to this as 'arising and passing'. This is a fundamental wisdom of many great spiritual teachings.

I ask clients to feel where their body is tight or uncomfortable and to inquire – what is the feeling here? It might be simply tightness, but the discomfort often has a tone to it. If a person has access to their emotions more readily, they may report that this area feels angry, frustrated, stifled, impatient or fearful. For some people, a visual image comes to mind, like a piece of tightly knotted rope or a steel brick. It may also have a texture or temperature, like burning hot sandpaper or freezing cold slippery ice, which the sensate types might find more readily comes to mind. This gives some access to the way in which our other senses relate to our emotions, giving them time and space to be explored. This way we are neither fully consumed by them to the point where it feels impossible to act in helpful ways, nor pushing them under the carpet. In short, we can have our emotions, instead of them 'having' us.

The practices in this chapter are not intended to replace counselling or psychotherapy, but can offer a link between body feeling and emotion, allowing a person to gain greater access to emotions so that they can be released or worked through.

Non-violent communication offers tools that can create more harmony in the emotional realm, when relationship to oneself and the outer world causes emotional friction that keeps us awake at night. This seeks to prevent the build-up of resentments and conflict that, over time, lead to emotional distress and sleeplessness. This method begins with identifying our own emotions and what has given rise to them, and helps us to be clear about what we need and want so that we can (a) meet our own needs, (b) negotiate with others to help us or (c) recognize that a situation will not be resolved in a way that meets our needs.

This and the self-management/meditation presented below operate on the basis of compassion for ourselves and acceptance of emotion. There are countless other techniques for managing emotion, and trained counsellors and therapists will have a range of skills and tools, as well as their relational presence. The tools mentioned here are offered as signposts for those who don't always deal with the emotional realms in practice but who wish to offer some ideas to their clients.

PRACTICE: EMOTIONAL CLEANSING BODY AWARENESS

Following on from the paragraphs above, this technique can help bring awareness to emotions. This helps us to no longer 'resist' emotion so that it no longer has to 'persist'. When we get to the emotional root of tension in the body, this can help us to ease into sleep more deeply. We can gain insight into something that's been beneath the surface of conscious awareness. Combined with a reflective practice, this meditation helps to get to the root reason for discomfort, pain or sabotage.

Step by Step

- Sit upright, comfortably, with your eyes closed, and breathe gently for 30 seconds. Become aware of your body.

- Feel the place in your body where you're holding the most tension.

- Ask yourself what feeling or tone is associated with that tightness. For example, you may be able to sense that it resembles impatience, anxiety, fear, anger or sadness.

- Breathe with awareness in the area.

- Say to yourself (in your head), as you inhale, 'I feel x', and then insert whatever the feeling is.

- On your exhale (and this is the revolutionary part) you say to yourself, again, in your head, 'I welcome x' or 'I accept x' or 'I allow x', and put in that same emotion.

- Stay with this for five to ten minutes or more.

- Notice any changes in the sensation and in the emotion you associate with it.

- Most often you will notice that the sensation and emotion may increase, change and eventually decrease.

- When the emotion shifts, the sensation may diminish or change location.

- If it changes location, stay with that area until you have felt-into and allowed the shifts to occur there.

Many people report greater insight into the link between their body-sensation and emotional state, and that this practice leaves them feeling freer and clearer.

Non-Violent Communication – the Yamas and Niyamas in Action

Marshall Rosenberg's books on non-violent communication (e.g. Rosenberg, 2003) provide a method for moving from hidden emotion to communication and solutions, which puts into action the non-violence principle found in the yamas and niyamas of the Yoga Sutras.

Non-violent communication is based on the idea that conflicts arise between people due to miscommunication about their human needs. When we feel discomfort, we can use coercive or manipulative language that aims to induce fear, guilt or shame in other people rather than accepting our emotions, working through them, asking for what we need from others, and resolving conflicts. Instead, non-violent communication seeks to help people clarify their needs, their feelings, their perceptions and their requests, thus minimizing conflict.

The emotional residue of unresolved conflict can result in playing out emotionally charged situations in our heads before sleep or in the middle of the night. We start by identifying our discomfort and what has given rise to it. Through meditation and the above body-based scan, we can learn to sit with the emotion long enough to work it through rather than shut it down or act out to avoid the discomfort. We then move to identifying the *needs* that it flags up, so that we can then seek to meet those needs within ourselves or in communication with others.

Part B: Emotions and Overwhelm: Overcoming Post-Traumatic Insomnia

If insomnia is a symptom of post-traumatic stress, the practices in the other sections of this programme may be helpful on their own, or may need to be adapted. It is possible that trauma is in play if the insomnia is accompanied by:

- anxiety

- phobias or unexplained fears

- severe mood swings, hyper-vigilance

- obsessions/compulsions

- physical symptoms that seem to have no medical diagnosis (chronic pain)

- difficulty learning and concentrating.

In terms of yoga therapy work, you may find that a client responds to yoga practices that are intended to create relaxation with panic, stress, dissociation or other paradoxical physical, mental or emotional reactions. This is a sign that a post-traumatic reaction may be in play.

Traumatic shock can be caused by an inescapable attack, physical injury/accident, war, natural disaster, birth trauma, severe abandonment or torture/abuse, as well as a variety of other causes, outlined in the following pages. This chapter discusses briefly three forms of post-trauma reaction, PTSD, developmental trauma and 'complex' PTSD, and offers some suggestions for your approach to yoga therapy for insomnia when trauma is an underlying factor in the sleep problems.

> **Marielle** looks fit and healthy in her late fifties, and leads a very active and artistic lifestyle. In our initial session, she disclosed that she wasn't always so well. She had been through treatment for breast cancer in her mid-forties, and it had been caught early enough for her to survive and thrive. Marielle doesn't appear anxious in the traditional sense, and is not aware of work problems or daily thoughts as she goes to bed. For her, sleep itself felt somehow scary: ever since her diagnosis she had trouble settling and letting go.
>
> After doing the pre-sleep yoga for two weeks she reported back that she found it easier to relax in the evening, and she was better able to notice that a sense of panic would set in just as her body started to drift off into sleep. She noticed that it was difficult for her to close her eyes in meditation, and that instead of relaxing her, it would cause her to feel more tense, and images from her time in hospital would flash into her mind. Given her history, I suggested that she see a trauma specialist to help her to repattern her response to 'going under' or 'letting go'.
>
> Marielle's response to major surgery and fear for her life remained long after the initial fright, and long after she was conscious of the response. Practising yoga helped, and her work in Somatic Experiencing (SE) therapy with a qualified practitioner helped her to de-activate the stress responses that prevented her from relaxing deeply in her yoga practice, and in her sleep. Even after she finished her SE sessions, Marielle kept pre-bed yoga and breath practices in place as part of her lifestyle, as they helped her enjoy the time before bed.

PTSD is Physiological, Mental and Emotional

The latest wave of theory and practice around trauma recovery acknowledges that post-traumatic stress disorder and other post-trauma disruptions in functioning involve embodied physiological states – not merely thoughts, emotions or states of mind. In the past 20 years, various practitioner-theorists have developed explanations for the mechanisms by which trauma is lodged in the body, brain and nervous system – and how we recover. The following is a general description, which is intended to assist you with identifying whether this may be in play with your yoga therapy for insomnia clients. After a brief explanation of what trauma is and contemporary understanding of how recovery from trauma works, I'll offer some ways to be more trauma-informed in yoga therapy for insomnia.

First, since shock trauma causes a physiological, biologically natural, response, its effect is not under mental, logical-rational control. For this reason, 'talk' counselling or psychotherapy may not resolve the symptoms, and some of the symptoms may show up in the body during yoga asana, breath work or meditation practice. In particular, practices that are intended to feel relaxing may cause stress responses rather than relaxation. Therefore, we may need to adapt the practices we offer.

Dr Peter Levine, in his books *Waking the Tiger* (1997) and *In an Unspoken Voice* (2010), notes how both humans' and wild animals' biological response systems become activated in response to perceived life-threatening situations. When overwhelmed by a threat where fight or flight is not possible, animals and humans enter into a freeze response (also known as immobility). Animals innately and quickly return to normal by allowing the involuntary mechanism that allows their nervous system to 'discharge' their excess survival energy and re-establish equilibrium. Levine's work illustrates how human beings often over-ride their instinctual systems, and block the involuntary discharge of the nervous system – due to societal and cultural constraints, we remain in a highly charged yet frozen state, much like a car with both the brakes and the accelerator floored simultaneously.

I interviewed Frances Ross, a UK-based trauma therapist, and practitioner of Levine's Somatic Experiencing model, who described how 'the nervous system must be allowed to resolve an unfinished pattern. Physiologically, humans are wired to go through the sequences of orientation and fight–flight when in a threatening situation.' When our natural ways of orientating and defending ourselves are blocked, this may cause us to experience one of two emotional states: rage (fight), and physiologically based terror panic (flight). It is the inability to flee or defend oneself that results in traumatic anxiety. Ross says that 'because physical sensation is the language of the instinctual brain, tracking the subtle body experience creates a natural opening for the involuntary release to occur. By guiding people gently into the realm of body sensation, somatic work helps them regain the ability to regulate their own nervous system.'

Different Types of PTSD and Their Impact
Developmental, Relational Trauma, Attachment and Security

Shock trauma has an impact on a person as he matures through the stages of development – from infancy, childhood and adolescence into adulthood. Developmental trauma may result from neglect and poor attunement or problems in attachment between child and caregiver. Frances Ross gives examples: a child abused within their family at an early age may not be able to form a secure attachment. A child hospitalized at an early age for prolonged periods may lose some of her sense of earlier successful attachment. These all affect the baseline level of security and safety, with corresponding impacts on the nervous system. A child who's been in danger during times of rest or sleep may never have learnt to rest comfortably and to relax enough to sleep well. Unless repaired, this pattern will persist into adulthood.

Complex PTSD

Complex post-traumatic stress disorder (CPTSD) was first described by Judith Herman in her book *Trauma and Recovery* (1992). Essentially, CPTSD involves a distortion and damage to a person's identity and sense of self. It is the result of persistent, prolonged abuse from a caregiver or in another close relationship. Situations that can give rise to CPTSD include sexual, emotional or physical abuse or neglect in childhood, domestic partner violence, being the victim of a kidnapping or hostage situation, suffering long-term work-related abuse (slavery, indentured servitude, human trafficking) or experience of concentration camps. These experiences can extend the feelings of terror, worthlessness and helplessness into other areas of life. For those who have experienced these types of trauma, it is understandable that sleep patterns, among many other rhythms, are likely to be disturbed and distorted.

A Yoga Therapy Approach to Post-Traumatic Insomnia

Below we look at two major ways in which trauma reactions can interact with yoga therapy for insomnia. We will then turn to an exploration of how the practices in this book relate to, and can be adapted to meet, the needs of those who are recovering from trauma-based insomnia.

As we have seen, a trauma response is the body–mind system's way of staying on alert to protect us from harm. This is functional when there is danger present. However, post-trauma disorders mean that the alarm bells are always switched on, or that they switch on in response to things we perceive through the senses: a specific sight, sound or smell can spark a memory or flashback. What may be 'nothing' to one person may be of great importance to a person with a trauma response to that sensory information.

As Judith Herman notes in her book, research tells us that traumatic events can actually *recondition the human nervous system, making sleep far less restful.* In people experiencing post-traumatic stress, increased nervous system arousal persists *during* sleep as well as in the waking state, resulting in numerous types of sleep disturbance. People with post-traumatic stress take longer to fall asleep, are more sensitive to noise and awaken more frequently during the night than those who aren't in post-traumatic stress. This makes sleep far less enjoyable, and the post-trauma experience may be compounded further by 'self-restricted sleep' or not going to bed because doing so is simply fraught with frustration.

In yoga therapy work I have observed the following:

1. **Sometimes 'relaxing' isn't relaxing:** In any group of more than ten people, I find at least one client may be unable to relax at the end of a yoga class, may seem deeply uncomfortable with breath practices, or may find it agitating to close their eyes in meditation. They may seem to fidget or space-out

in a therapy session, or may carry intense muscle tension during a massage.

I have seen several clients who are desperate for relaxation techniques, but as soon as they drop down into relaxation the sense of panic, a jolt or reactivation occurs. Relaxation itself can feel so unsafe, due to life events, that relaxation techniques or the sensation of relaxation incites panic or tension. When a person in a post-traumatic pattern begins to relax into the early stages of sleep, as the initial exhaustion of the homeostatic drive towards sleep diminishes, or during the brain activity of REM sleep, they may awaken with a racing heart, fast breath or anxious thoughts. They may experience nightmares or night terrors.

A client may present with a fear or anxiety response to sleep, or to life events more broadly. Perhaps none of the thinking-or-talking-based analytical solutions or none of the medical and behavioural solutions seem to have dislodged his sleep problems.

2. **Fear of sleep can cause sleep sabotage:** Some of my clients know what they 'should' do but their sleep habits are consistently sabotaged by addictive or compulsive actions. I have some clients who fear nightmares and the distress caused by sleep due to trauma, so they drink alcohol or take sedatives to get to sleep. These forms of coping don't repair the underlying cause of the insomnia, they stop working quickly, and often have detrimental effects on their mental state the next day. Others still stay up very late, avoiding sleep until they are totally exhausted, and don't leave enough time for a night's sleep before they need to be awake. This often combines with middle-of-night awakening, when the activation in the nervous system over-rides the homeostatic drive towards sleep. This perpetuates a vicious cycle of sleeplessness.

Recovery from trauma-based insomnia relies on the individual either relearning or repatterning their response to sleep and relaxation, or learning for the first time (as in the case of very early trauma) the capacity to self-soothe. In addition to discharging the aroused, heightened state as described above, what's needed is the *repair* of the sense of safety. Repairing, or establishing for the first time, feelings of safety and comfort decreases the urge to escape, numb or self-medicate that spur sleep-sabotaging habits such as alcohol and drug abuse, and other addictive behaviours that can cause or exacerbate insomnia. As Frances Ross states it, 'therapist and client work together to develop a core within himself to which he can attach, or a "resource" for safety rather than attaching to people and things outside of himself'. This sense of internal safety extends into sleep patterns, making it easier to release into sleep – feeling secure enough to stay asleep.

The following draws on my clinical experience, and upon the written work of David Emerson (2015) and Dagmar Härle (2017). It is intended to help you to:

1. tailor your approach to yoga therapy for insomnia in ways that are more trauma-informed

2. seek further training

3. refer onward to an appropriate practitioner, or resources, with an understanding of what you are helping the client to seek out.

Listen for the Signs: The Intake

I've learnt to listen carefully during an initial client session, taking a basic history of a person's sleep problems. It's useful to know if the problem can be traced back to a memorable event or a particular time period, or whether they say, 'I have never been a good sleeper', with sleep problems dating back to childhood or teen years. However, there are many reasons that a client might *not* include traumatic experiences on an intake form or when you're taking their history. Some of this information may come out as you work together over several sessions. Why might a client neglect to mention that they have experienced a traumatic event or events?

- Your client may not feel it appropriate – or safe – to disclose the deeper dynamics of family history or past events. There may be feelings of guilt or shame – or fear of judgement – that inhibits them from disclosing an abuse or other trauma.

- Your client may not see the links between long-ago occurrences and their inability to sleep today – they may not see it as relevant without a prompt.

- For some people, there is no memory of traumatic events. Memories may be held back from conscious awareness because they are too painful to experience in the here-and-now.

- Traumatizing events like abuse or neglect may be remembered but may have been normalized. This can be part of an abuse pattern – 'normalizing' the abusive practices or behaviour.

To Recover Good Sleep...or Find It for the First Time?

Even if a person doesn't disclose a traumatic event, it's possible to understand post-trauma insomnia as it relates to a person's history. If there was a pattern of good sleep at some point, recovery becomes a process of restoring. If there was never a resource of pleasant, restful sleep, it may be a matter of your client establishing an entirely new set of experiences.

Post-Traumatic Stress Disorder: 'I used to sleep OK before'

If traumatic events were preceded by a good-enough set of formative childhood experiences, a client will have previously experienced the mental and physical sensations of safety, relaxation and healthy sleep. If a person then experiences a severe trauma, it is possible that they can 'return' to a state of relaxation that they once knew. A more instructional or directive approach may be possible and useful for them. In this case, learning yoga practices can help the individual to self-regulate (release tension or create wakefulness) and to reintroduce relaxation bit by bit. Marielle, described earlier, shows this type of post-traumatic sleep problem.

Early, Complex or Relational Trauma: 'I've never been a good sleeper'

If a person has experienced abuse, neglect or attack early in life, in the home, you may hear things like 'I've never been a good sleeper' or 'I've always avoided sleep' or 'I don't really like to sleep but feel exhausted all the time'. For them, sleep may never have been a refuge: it may have been a prelude to predation or a time of great vulnerability to attack. If the life events led to complex or relational trauma, going to sleep may involve feelings of terror, overwhelm, being overpowered and being subject to force or coercion, restraint or manipulation. It may be the case that the person's body, mind and psyche never learnt safety, relaxation and healthy sleep, and that the things associated with powerlessness and letting go are inherently scary. Lina's example in this book shows this type of post-traumatic insomnia.

Identifying Trauma's Effects

According to Peter Levine, the response to attack, abuse or threat may display in several physiological ways and he offers a 'long list' of additional symptoms of trauma in three layers or sets, in an accessible small book for laypeople (Levine, 2008). These may relate to things your client feels and experiences in their day-to-day life.

1. More direct trauma symptoms include difficulty sleeping, hypervigilance, intrusive imagery or flashbacks, extreme sensitivity to light or noise, hyperactivity, an exaggerated startle response, nightmares or night terrors, abrupt mood swings (tantrums, rage, outbursts), shame and lack of self-worth, and reduced ability to deal with stress (chronically stressed out).

2. Trauma response may also show up as amnesia, panic attacks or blankness, avoidance of certain situations, attraction to dangerous situations, addictions, exaggerated or diminished sexual activity, inability to love or form attachments, fear of dying or a shortened life, self-mutilation, or loss of sustaining (spiritual or moral) beliefs.

3. In the longer term, post-trauma responses may involve 'retracting from life': shyness, diminished emotional responses,

inability to make commitments or form plans, depression. It may also involve 'longer term stress-related ailments' due to chronic sympathetic nervous system arousal breaking down hormonal balance: chronic fatigue, immune system problems, psychosomatic illnesses, chronic pain, fibromyalgia, asthma, skin disorders, digestive disorders, severe PMS/PMT.

With Levine's descriptions of the underlying physiological causes of trauma symptoms, we can understand how different trauma-related states can be affected by yoga practices that may help to alleviate or recondition these responses in the longer term. These may not be immediate effects, and in the case of complex trauma, as outlined below, it may be best to offer non-directive options rather than instruction.

Hyper-arousal: increased heart rate and breath rate, sweating, etc., as described in the section on sympathetic arousal. Breath awareness or practice can decrease the arousal in the nervous system. Bringing gentle attention to, and eventually slowing down, the rate of breathing can increase one's confidence in feelings of safety. When a person begins to feel and sense that a more relaxed state is within her reach through the breath, this capacity grows over time as a resource upon which to draw if a trigger is activated. For example, if a person feels the panic rising, it may become easier over time to decrease the physiological response if a person has the ability to alter her breathing.

Constriction in the body occurs in a post-traumatic response; with narrowing of perception, internal organs constrict and the digestive system is inhibited. To counter the sensation of narrowed perception, when tightening occurs, a person may begin to make use of breath and movement slowly, with her own internal sense of rhythm. This can create a growing sense of ease and expansion. Increasing a sense of relaxation and focus while moving or pressing outward to lengthen the muscles can de-constrict and expand the physical musculature. Gentle movement, for example in twisting postures, can also bring greater movement around, and perhaps circulation to the viscera and internal organs.

Dissociation relates to the secretion of endorphins (as Levine calls them, 'nature's internal opium') to numb the pain associated with attack. Endorphins can help a person endure experiences that they otherwise may not have been able to bear. This results in what Herman and Levine call 'fragmentation': a part of the body feels disconnected from awareness or numb. A person may also experience feeling separate from, or outside of, themselves.

Yoga practices can bring sensation back into the body in a safe environment. In therapeutic yoga we move consciously, connecting body and brain, attending to the sensation. Sometimes it's helpful to connect with the movement as the student watches, for example, their foot stepping back or uses self-touch, for example pressing their own hand onto their hamstring as it stretches. Connecting visual, physical sensation and movement can help a person to re-establish a sense of connection.

Denial is not something that people do intentionally. Shock is a state of overwhelm in which one is not able to take in that the event has occurred. A greater capacity for noticing body sensations (interoception) can provide a person with clues to their mental state, helping them to re-access their present time reality, and own feelings of overwhelm before they cause shut-down. This can in turn help a person to tolerate difficult and overwhelming experiences so that they may become more conscious, can be processed, and released.

Feelings of helplessness, immobility and freezing. Moving the body at one's own will, creating forms and gaining strength can help create feelings of efficacy and agency. For example, being able to hold in a Warrior position may help a person to create feelings of strength and increasing stability.

A yoga therapy-based insomnia recovery approach can involve a person developing feelings of bodily integrity, agency and safety slowly, over time. A trauma-sensitive or non-directive yoga approach is particularly recommended here.

Asana: Trauma Considerations

For some people who experience PTSD, the yoga postures in the previous chapters may be of use in re-establishing connection between body and mind. Some clients find instruction and alignment cues useful in directing attention to the various parts of their body, especially if there is no general numbing or dissociation. The general approach to yoga therapy for insomnia in this book is based on clear instruction of generally useful methods, and providing support for these practices, either one to one or in groups. After instruction, the majority of practice is self-practice.

In the initial teaching phase it's essential for student and teacher to note any adverse reactions to the postures or practices. Each person who experiences PTSD can have different symptoms, which may make some yoga movements problematic, while others may feel extremely soothing. For the purpose of relaxing at bedtime, I have found the sequences – the Simple Sleep Sequence and Deeper Sleep Sequence – can be adapted to what the practitioner finds safe and pleasant.

I offer the client a preview of the postures, whether they prefer for me to demonstrate the movement, or prefer to see a printed chart or stick figure drawing of what I'm suggesting. The client can point out any postures that seem problematic. These can be avoided, or I can offer alternative stretches. I suggest moving into postures slowly to note any signs of distress related to any of the movements. I'll say 'this is another option' and give a variation on the theme. For those with complex trauma due to bodily attacks or relational trauma, it's important to watch out for the following things.

Movements may trigger '**bodily recall**' – image flashbacks or distressing body sensation that emerges when in a particular position or movement. Some students may be aware of the effect of a pose and avoid it. Others may feel subtle pressure to 'perform' the pose (even if your instruction allows for variation or skipping it). If the student does the pose, she may simultaneously self-protect internally by dis-associating, sending awareness out of the body. This may look like the person has 'checked out' with eyes upward or glazed in a form of shut-down. It may also arise as shaking or convulsing involuntarily in a posture or practice. If this occurs it is useful to approach quietly and to speak gently to help the person come back to the present moment and back into a present-time sensation such as the feeling of their feet on the floor.

Emerson (2015) and Härle's (2017) work indicates that experiencing early and/or severe abuse at the hands of another person may mean that the **directive nature of teaching** or instructing specific yoga asana or practices can establish an unhelpful power dynamic. Those with complex trauma experiences may have heightened sensitivity to performing according to others' wishes or expectations. It is important to avoid re-creating, even on a subtle level, a situation in which the client feels her body is subject to another person's control, demands, evaluation or judgement. This is difficult to do while maintaining complex postures with safety instructions for alignment. For those who have experienced early bodily manipulation or control, there may be a pattern of over-riding one's own internal cues in standard practice of yoga postures in order to 'do the pose correctly'. By contrast, it can be reparative and empowering to be offered possibilities for movement by invitation and by choice, without standards to be achieved or forms to be attained. Specifically 'trauma-sensitive yoga' as taught by the Boston-based Trauma Center (referred to as TCTSY, or Trauma Center Trauma Sensitive Yoga) is invitational, exploratory and largely non-directive in nature.

For example, Emerson (2015) describes the use of 'muscle dynamics', which involves sensing the movement and quality of muscular experiences such as lengthening and contracting, noticing shifts in intensity, adding purpose to movement, and using one's own hand to touch the moving musculature. These are ways of developing 'interoception', or the ability to sense within one's own body, rather than taking a particular shape to achieve a goal. This internal direction creates the conditions necessary for a person to 'take effective action' on her own behalf to adjust to internal and external circumstances. Emerson (2015) and Härle's (2017) books and the corresponding training programmes offer extensive support for providing options.

Pranayama: Trauma Considerations

For those who experience hyper-arousal, it can be very difficult to engage in any techniques that control or direct the breath. Strong or 'elevating' pranayama can cause difficulty, especially for those who have experienced shock-trauma such as bomb blasts, have been attacked in ways that inhibited their breath, or for people who experience panic attacks. Breath retention (holding after the in-breath on 'full' or after the out-breath on 'empty' or anywhere in between) is not advised in these circumstances.

David Emerson's work suggests an open and exploratory and non-directive approach to breath when working with those who have experienced complex trauma. In fact TCTSY does not teach pranayama *per se* but attention to the breath and bodily sensations that surround it, again developing interoceptive awareness. Unlike the breath practices in this book, TCTSY doesn't practise breathing for a purpose – in order to energize or to relax. In the TCTSY model, breathing is seen as 'just another way to experience the dynamic possibilities that having a body entails; to notice what we feel; and to make some choices'. TCTSY works with 'dynamic qualities of the breath' to offer opportunities for clients to have 'new body experiences that may be different from trauma, if that trauma limits or constrains our capacity to breathe in some way' (Emerson, 2015).

Trauma Considerations with Marma, Meditation and Mantra

Self-acupressure may be helpful as a way to begin to connect breath with physical sensation for those who experience body numbing. I have used these with clients who are seeking an alternative to self-harming behaviours, and I work with them to ensure that healthy moderation is used in applying pressure. Some evidence suggests that self-harming mobilizes endorphin responses to pain, and as noted in the section of this book dealing with marma points, this is said to be the same mechanism through which acupressure works.

There are widely noted benefits of meditation as outlined in this book, and many of these can extend to people who have experienced trauma. However, those who are experiencing post-traumatic stress *may* find the relaxation at the end of yoga classes or given as part of a yoga therapy course difficult or even impossible. For some people, closing their eyes doesn't feel safe, and a person may have more or less distress lying on their back or seated upright, depending upon the individual. Closing the eyes or lying down for 'relaxation' can set off a response from 'fidgety' to flashbacks to a sense of panic. Depending upon the person and her experience, this may occur when the person is alone, in a one-to-one setting, or in a group. Evidence suggests that while people with non-traumatized responses shift from Beta brain waves (active) to Alpha brain waves (relaxed) upon closing their eyes, those with PTSD experience heightened Beta waves upon closing their eyes. For those who experience difficulty practising relaxation techniques with eyes closed, it is often useful to attempt these with eyes open or possibly down-cast to look at the floor or yoga mat. Increasing tolerance to eyes-closed relaxation without force or rush can help a person to increase feelings of safety during sleep times.

For post-traumatic insomnia clients, mantra repeated internally with eyes closed may also be difficult. In this case, chanting, singing or making sound may be a useful practice. Evidence suggests that singing and chanting provide additional therapeutic benefits such as toning of the vagus nerve, which in turn makes a person more adaptive to stress, and less reactive. It's useful to be aware that chanting can be triggering for those who have experienced certain types of religious or ritualistic abuse – it is always vital to check in with a client and note their reactions to the suggestion of a practice.

Becoming More Trauma-Informed in Group Classes

In my yoga for insomnia group classes and courses, there is a broad range of students, ranging from those who have never done any yoga before to experienced yoga teachers. In teaching yoga for insomnia, it's important to be aware that a proportion of the students will have had insomnia as a trauma response. It's best to incorporate some sensitivity to this in these classes. The following are based on my own experience, and I drew upon a helpful article by Linda Karl in *Yoga Therapy Today* (2012).

Environment

Making the environment as safe and predictable as possible can enable greater relaxation and avoid triggers. It can be hard for a trauma survivor to relax if he feels the room is not secure, for example an open door, having one's back to the door, people entering the room unexpectedly, too much or too little light in the room and sudden noises are best avoided if possible. In some of my classes, a fan on a timer goes off at a certain time. I usually give notice that this will happen and indicate that it's normal to feel a little startle when it does. If I forget to mention it, when the noise does occur, I explain what it is, note that a startle response is common, and offer the possibility of lengthening the exhale and feeling the body's connection to the floor to promote feelings of safety.

Language

Concise, directional language is very valuable in standard yoga instruction. A trauma-sensitive approach, however, generally avoids phrases that sound controlling, and favours self-empowerment. To teach in a way that helps with insomnia recovery, it helps to pace your instructions slowly. Pause after a cue so that the student can integrate it. Some methods, including Emerson's (2015) work, use repetition of the cues, so that if a student or client has checked-out momentarily, they are given ample opportunity to re-engage. Trauma-sensitive cues emphasize choice – about when to move and to what extent, encouraging students to move in ways that feel safer; even if a stretch feels strong, a sense of safety is vital.

Language that emphasizes self-inquiry and attention to one's own body sense – rather than performance or accomplishment – is helpful in increasing the self-soothing capacity needed to get to sleep and manage wake-ups in the middle of the night.

In particular where complex trauma and other relational traumas are present, beginning a cue with language such as 'I want you to do x' or 'Do x for me' may be particularly triggering. These cues may subtly infuse a sense of another person's will over the student's experience or movement. These cues are best avoided, as we are seeking to promote the student's own bodily choices and movement.

Assisting and Touch

The use of touch in yoga classes may be very comforting to some students, while for others it can be distressing. Even watching a teacher touch someone else might raise doubts about safety. In general, it helps to minimize physical assists, restricting them to the essentials and using verbal cues if at all possible – for example, 'If you move your heel forward to just underneath your knee in this lunge, it will take the strain off your knee.' This helps a student to learn a movement for herself. This also promotes verbal skill and clarity in the teacher, respects the student's bodily integrity and helps her to align her own body, integrating the movement for her own use later.

Guidelines for Physical Adjustments

Here are some guidelines I use for physical adjustments, to be sensitive to the possibility of trauma in my students:

- Be clear internally about the intention behind any physical assists, and don't offer them unless a clear rapport has been established with the student.

- Ask permission and give a sense of what you are offering: 'May I assist you to twist a bit more in your upper back?'

- Outline what you are offering verbally first: 'This means I'll help you stabilize your back and I'll place a hand on your shoulder-blade – is that OK?' I will often move my hands to show the direction of the assist so that the student can see the action and make a choice.

- Move with care, firmly and succinctly, and if the person looks distressed, stop.

- If you happen to brush a sensitive area unintentionally, acknowledge it immediately so that it's clear it was not intentional – for example, 'I'm sorry for the unintentional [boob, butt, leg] touch.' It can be an awkward situation, so a sense of clarity and even humour can help.

Above all things: keep it clear and conscious.

Choice of Physical/Asana Practices

Some people find a slow flow comforting, while others feel more stable in long holds in static positions, particularly standing poses. Some people find lying on their back on the floor soothing, while others find it disconcerting or distressing. A slow class with some repetition can be comforting, and a slower pace can allow awareness to settle in the body.

It is important to note that, where there has been sexual trauma, rotating the legs open to expose the genital area can feel scary or humiliating. Strong chest openers and back-bends may evoke powerful bodily sensations and heightened emotions. In her article in *Yoga Therapy Today*, Karl (2012) suggests introducing postures slowly and incrementally, bringing in a new pose with familiar poses before and after. Consistency can also feel comforting, so teaching the same sequences for a period of time can be useful. This is my experience with the Simple Sleep Sequence – repetition and familiarity breed comfort and safety when the poses are not triggering. For some students who prefer not to lie down supine, the Deeper Sleep Sequence offers more upright alternatives to several poses.

Managing an Unexpected Reaction in a Group Class

Unexpected reactions may be disconcerting for student and teacher, but it's important to understand that this may be a way of managing conscious or unconscious anxiety.

In this case it is helpful to quietly offer the student some alternatives:

1. Another option for a movement that the student prefers – you can offer one or two suggestions particularly, activating the large muscles of the body. If a stress response occurs, it can sometimes help to invite the student to start moving the large muscles in the legs (for example, in the Warrior or other standing poses done dynamically). It is thought that those muscles use up the stress hormone cortisol. For some students, focusing on the breath to calm the nervous system can be helpful.

2. Sitting comfortably, if the student is more comfortable with the support of a wall behind the back, or in Child's Pose if appropriate.

3. Taking time out of the room if needed to manage overwhelm – it's helpful to have a specific place and possibly to encourage the student to come back as and when they feel ready.

Offering Resources and Referrals

If you aren't a qualified psychotherapist yourself, it is highly recommended that you find a good referral for clients who may benefit from trauma work. For this, I recommend working with a practitioner with a long-term psychotherapeutic qualification and licensed status with membership in a reputable professional association in addition to trauma-related training. Therapists are trained in the nuances of the therapeutic relationship or 'container' for working at depth. Accredited psychotherapy programmes develop sensitivity and skill in the relationship of client to therapist, look at how to manage attachment and boundaries, and offer structures for supervision and oversight of therapists. It may also feel safer and more confidential to see another practitioner, rather than disclosing personal information to you, especially if you see them in group settings or busy yoga studios.

Chapter Five

The Soul

Sleeplessness as a Call to Awaken

For a person to heal truly, rather than just alleviate symptoms, there needs to be a *transformation*, which underlies the movement from unwellness to wellness. At the core of this programme is the idea that recovery involves the *life force* of a person. Whether you choose to call it their soul or spirit, or something else, healing involves it. Healing can be called a spiritual practice in that it starts with an intention to be well, and a desire to put an end to the suffering that's caused by being unwell. Some people might call this intention a prayer – we can translate that intention into a treatment plan. A path towards healing begins to form as soon as a person decides to seek help, and you can assist them as soon as you are engaged in the process with them.

As healers, practitioners and clinicians, we hear their desire to heal, and assist that process as best we can. It's said that *prayer* is a process of articulating what is longed for and asking for it – from life, nature, a higher power, the divine or God – and that *meditation* is the process of diving into stillness and quiet to listen for answers, intuition, guidance and truth. As we help others to heal we can facilitate both of these processes, especially if we can engage with them ourselves in our own lives. It doesn't matter whether you or your clients are agnostic, atheist, Christian, Muslim, Jewish, Hindu or any other faith. Yoga as a healing modality invites you to call it what you will, but to use the positive healing potential of the life force, on all levels, to restore wellness. Along the way, we have the opportunity to build our awareness, to learn new tools and skills, to mourn losses, to celebrate progress and to become more full-spectrum human beings. It is a great gift, to learn how to heal ourselves and others.

When we engage with another person towards healing, we need this capacity to hear their longing, and to listen to what they present to help them find their answers. We hear the call, and assist with the response.

What's Keeping Us Awake May Be 'Awakening' Us

It is possible that sleep recovery can be unlocked when we find the right key: some combination of yogic practices, sleep hygiene-related habit change, emotional outlet or mind management techniques may restore good sleep. The tools and techniques I've presented in each chapter of this book so far can resolve a great deal, when presented clearly and invitingly as part of a course, or when a skilled therapist and client work together one on one, crafting an intelligent and elegant healing path. At other times, the knowledge, tools and techniques in the previous chapters aren't enough, and sleep is still elusive – your client is literally restless. When this is the case, we need to look at that restlessness more closely, to hear what it's saying to us. We need to heed the alarm-call of sleeplessness, and realize that something within is both keeping that person awake, and is serving to 'wake up' that person.

This final chapter takes as its inspiration the name of the inner layer of the five-kosha system, the anandamaya kosha, translated as the 'bliss' body. While spiritual traditions acknowledge that life involves suffering, the invitation of the five koshas is to move both towards and from something the ancients called 'bliss'. This is different from a personality that's happy-all-the-time. It is something more pervasive, related to a form of consciousness that is continuous with the infinite nature of the self. Put simply, this means we are more than our bodies, our circulation, our mind and our emotions – we are something that can witness all of this as a form of consciousness, *and* we are both connected to, and a part of, a vitality and power-source that is lifelong, and may exist beyond our lifetime. Some call this the soul or spirit, some call it a connection to God, the divine, the universe or nature. The purpose of this chapter is not to define what spirituality means for you or for your clients, but to point to this 'inner layer' of ourselves as vital to our overall and abiding wellness.

A Non-Dogmatic, Spiritual Dimension of Yoga Therapy

Rather than a reductionist parts-to-whole approach, a yoga therapy perspective invites us to look at people as spiritual beings, connected by a universal life force, or *nature*. This may seem esoteric but is in fact very palpable, important and vital. As this approach to yoga therapy is inclusive of many traditions, we draw upon guidance from many sources. The Vietnamese Buddhist teacher Thich Nhat Hanh (2016) describes very practically the importance of a spiritual understanding in life. He says, 'Everyone needs a spiritual dimension in life... If we have this capacity, then we can develop real and lasting spiritual intimacy with ourselves and others.' The tenderness with which we listen to our own human needs, urges and longings, as well as attending to the needs of our bodies, living in alignment with the rhythm of day and night, can become parts of a *spiritual* practice. These form a kind of intimacy that honours the self and one's place in the world.

Hanh believes that:

> without a spiritual dimension, it's very challenging to be with the daily difficulties we all encounter. With a spiritual practice you're no longer afraid. Along with your physical body, you have a spiritual body. The practices of breathing, walking, concentration and understanding can help you greatly in dealing with your emotions, in listening to and embracing your suffering, and in helping you to recognize and embrace the suffering of another person. (p.32)

Throughout the millennia, spiritual practice has also served the purpose of instilling and supporting in human beings a sense of trust in nature or the process of life. It helps to address the fear of death that sits beneath much of our human inability to let go. This can be essential to the process of sleeping well.

But what do we mean by spirituality, exactly? Hahn points out what it isn't as a way to help clarify: spirituality 'doesn't mean a blind belief in a spiritual teaching. Spirituality is a *practice* that brings relief, communication, and transformation.' Yoga therapy, when viewed as the stewardship of a soul or spirit embodied, brings the following things:

- relief – in the form of alleviating tension, pain and agitation

- communication – in the form of dialogue with symptoms and our habits

- transformation in the form of lasting changes created over time in our bodies, minds and orientation to our lives.

Brian, the author we met earlier who initially appeared like an emaciated vampire with dull skin and sunken eyes, began with yoga postures that reanimated his body and colourized his form. He could then sit comfortably and took to meditation like a duck to water once tension and tightness in his body abated and he could sit comfortably. His sense of settling into himself was palpable. He began to feel relief – his sleep improved dramatically in a matter of weeks and he was able to get to sleep and mostly stay asleep for six to seven hours per night.

As mentioned in the Introduction, I ran into Brian on a commuter train several years after our course of yoga therapy and meditation. He's continued to meditate and uses yoga postures when he feels the need. He asked me about honeymoon recommendations: he and the girlfriend with whom he wouldn't move in during his acute insomnia were about to be married. When I contacted him about this book nearly two years after we bumped into each other, he told me, 'I'm sleepless again, but for entirely different, very happy reasons. I'm a dad now.' He's been in conversation with the challenges in his life, and recognized that he has the tools to handle them. He not only cured himself of his paralysing insomnia, but feels confident enough in managing his sleep that he has created a family with the woman he loves, with faith that he can handle it. This is indeed a profound transformation: Brian knows that he has the tools and resilience to recover from sleeplessness and not only to manage his days, but to 'take life on' fully.

This is very different from how modern approaches to sleep view the human being. A doctor might have put Brian on sleeping pills or given him a habit-based CBT approach, which would have been likely to keep Brian in his head, where he spent most of his time to begin with. Seeing him as a whole, understanding where his 'energy', circulation and balance needed to be refocused, unlocked not only his sleep, but also his sense of settled-ness into a life that not only held his work, but also growing love and connection.

An Alternative to Modern Machine Metaphors

Modern Western medicine teaches its physicians to break down a problem into its component parts to try to work out what is broken, deficient or diseased so that they can mend the broken part, or put in the right solvents or solutions, like a mechanic runs a diagnostic test to see what has caused a car to break down, finds the broken part and fixes it or replaces it, maybe putting in brake fluid or oil. Medical specialization divides the human system into manageable pieces, like the endocrine system, the muscles and bones, the ear/nose/throat, or the reproductive organs. This honing in is useful for many illnesses and disorders, although the reason that these disorders occur is often something far more pervasive, having to do with organic as well as psychological factors, as well as many inexplicable forces involved in governing who falls ill and who heals.

Brian came into the clinic describing his problems with sleep: 'I need to learn how to switch off.' Lina wished she could just 'find the right button to press to make the nightmares stop'. Simon suffered from panic attacks, and wanted to know how to 'shut down his mind'. It's not surprising that we're looking for mechanical quick fixes when we define the problem in this way. In a sense, this is how we have been taught to view ourselves by a diagnose-and-fix model of medicine, a machine metaphor that takes away the mystery of our humanity because it may feel unmanageable.

By contrast, the yoga tradition views us as not merely 'on' or 'off', but as capable of sliding in and out of different states of consciousness. While some people may appear to switch from 'on' to 'off' as they fall asleep quickly and easily, there is a process in which they move from a waking state through a twilight, drifting state, into sleep that can be faster or slower for each of us. If you have ever seen another living creature sleep, you can see that sleep involves patterns – faster or shallower breaths, total stillness or twitching limbs, a relaxed face or eyes moving beneath closed lids. We are anything but completely 'off'.

While we are alive, our power source is never gone. Instead, we move from one state of consciousness to another, with corresponding physical states. This is entirely different from what happens when we pull the plug on a machine or press a button to shut it down. A machine that's 'off' does not process anything and can't repair itself without power. A self-cleaning oven must be 'on' to do its work. A computer that is in standby mode may be able to carry out some anti-virus scans, but nothing happens when a machine is *off*. Perhaps our sleeplessness has become an epidemic because we expect ourselves to switch off like machines instead of being more expert in managing different states of our own human consciousness.

Simon didn't need to just shut off his mind, but to listen to it, and to his emotional world, as well as his body and how he spent his energy. It took having panic attacks for Simon to truly 'wake up'. He had tolerated chronic insomnia for as long as he could remember, and a trip to the hospital meant that he had to start taking his health and mental state very seriously. As we unravelled what had led him to his acute distress, the death of a close friend brought up his own fears of mortality, and many losses early in life. Working through yoga poses and breath practices enabled him to slow down and feel his fears, and gave him a sense of comfort in talking about things he found difficult. The poses put him in touch with when, during the day, he'd feel tension. The breath practices helped him notice when he'd tense up – shallower breath, higher heart rate, and a sense of floating above the ground. He learnt to take his nervous system out of high-alert through conscious breathing with longer exhalations. His daily meditation gave him time that he called 'executive time' to process not only his business dealings, but his family and inner world, so that he could respond instead of being reactive, and he found he saved a lot of time, taking more thoughtful action. Simon has softened – there is less heat and pressure in his world. He walks a little more slowly, but his strides are longer. His eyes are calmer: instead of protruding from his skull, they sparkle as he delivers his trademark jokes. He reveals more of his thoughts, feelings and inner world to a trusted inner circle of friends and family – he no longer hides behind a facade of intense activity achievement and sharp humour. He has become more effective in his business dealings, delegating more, with a keener sense of how he needs to spend his own time, and has continued his political work while minimizing the aspects of it that used to affect his sleep. He's clearer on his priorities, more sensitive to his needs, and more effective – with less strain and more joy.

Sleep and States of Consciousness

The ancient yogis recognized that consciousness has different forms, and gave names to these different states (Feuerstein, 2014; Olivelle, 1998):

- The awake state (jagrata) involves outward knowing and awareness of the gross world, including tangible things, and physical and external phenomena. When we are awake we can see and hear, taste and smell, touch, converse, and interact with people, places and things. In this state things are tangible.

- Dream-filled sleep (svapna) is when stuff you've perceived in your life comes back to you and is 'organized' by the unconscious. It doesn't follow the rules of the tangible, concrete world but offers fragments and symbols.

- Deep, dreamless sleep (susupti) is called the 'causal' layer in which nothing is 'doing' or playing in consciousness in terms of senses but consciousness is there, quiet. Perhaps it is a state of pure 'being'.

- The beyond-deep-sleep state (turiya) is the state to which committed yogis, often found in ashrams and on mountaintops, aspire. I'm not sure I have had personal experience of this state, so I can't share much about it from that perspective. For many people working and living in the world of transactions, interactions and getting and spending, realizing pure universal consciousness as not separate from all other beings or God may be a difficult task, while for others, 'non-dual awareness' is a reality.

Lina made changes in her sleeping environment and all of her life habits, but the most important change was in her ability to 'drop in' to rest physically – this gave her feelings of greater safety that permeated every aspect of her life. During the time we worked together she moved from feeling terror at the sensation of releasing her muscles and coming into rest, to shuddering as she did so, to being able to glide into relaxation more easily with each passing week. She took her nightmares back into therapy where she is working on them again: having had the experience of relaxing her body she is better able to confront her fears and has begun to feel more 'safe' in her skin. Since childhood she had always feared sleep because of the vulnerability it entailed, and the exposure to the risk of attack. Even *starting* to relax had felt unsafe for her and sleep was a minefield. Beginning with yoga postures, in which she was in control of her own body, helped her to assess the tension and relaxation in her muscles – she developed 'interoception' slowly, and has begun to feel what her body needs – food, rest, sleep, stretching – and be able to meet these. The missing piece for her was connecting her need for safety in her body that would build slowly over time. She feels safer in her skin, less afraid of harm or death as she goes into sleep and dreaming, knowing that she will be OK or that, if she experiences pain or distress, she can get help.

At the start of her course of yoga therapy sessions, she was smoking cigarettes, using coffee to manage her daytime exhaustion and working out in the gym to the point of collapse. She was sick of being single after a long-term relationship had broken up and felt that another relationship would be impossible. As Lina dropped into her body, she made changes to her diet that were more nourishing, gained weight that made her look calmer and healthier, and has begun noticing people more, establishing easier friendships and slowly opening up to the possibility of dating. Her work has become more enjoyable, and she finds herself laughing and smiling more heartily, feeling less afraid, sleeping better, and feeling more alive in her life.

The Chakra System, Waking Up and Alchemical Transformation

During the course of a day our energy is bounded. We may try to over-ride sleepiness, but can find ourselves in a state of depletion. The realization that we have a finite, yet replenishable, energy source is a vital part of sleep recovery and waking up during our days.

There is an elegant system that helps us to understand balance within the different aspects of ourselves. When one part of our personality and experience comes more to the foreground, other aspects recede. When we are imbalanced towards excess in some areas of life, we may be left short, or deficient, in other areas.

The modern understanding of the chakra system as put forward by body–mind therapist Anodea Judith in her foundational work *Wheels of Life* (1987) gives us a therapeutic and compassionate way to view the various aspects of the human system.

The word 'chakra' (pronounced with a 'ch' as in chocolate) is Sanskrit for 'wheel or disc' and signifies one of seven basic energy centres in the body that correspond to nerve ganglia branching out from the spinal column or organs/glands. These centres, from a body–mind psychospiritual perspective, relate to aspects of our lives – consciousness, developmental stages of life, archetypal elements, body functions, colours, sounds and more.

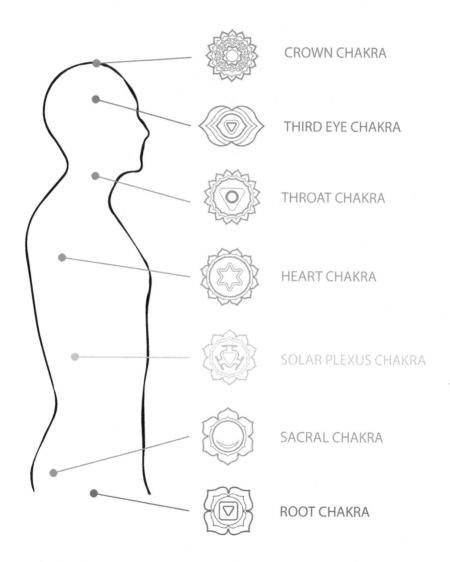

CROWN CHAKRA

THIRD EYE CHAKRA

THROAT CHAKRA

HEART CHAKRA

SOLAR PLEXUS CHAKRA

SACRAL CHAKRA

ROOT CHAKRA

The chakra system forms a map of different aspects of the human being, offering a way to view ourselves as a whole and providing a template for transformation. Judith's classic East–West integrative text *Wheels of Life* explores all of these inter-related aspects of the chakras. The system of chakras is said to be extensive throughout the body, and the number of primary chakras varies depending on the philosophical system or text. While some authors dispute the historical veracity of the system being explained here, it can be looked at as indicative – a way to begin a conversation about holistic balance to help ourselves and our clients back to good sleep and alert, awake days.

The lower chakras relate to aspects of bodily stability, relationship and will, while the upper chakras relate to love, expression, insight and spiritual connection. One way of understanding the movement from 'lower' to 'higher' aspects of the self is to call it a *'liberating'* current – one that takes the material and puts it into a bigger, more spiritual context. And moving from the 'higher' or more subtle aspects of self can be seen as grounding or bringing spirit into form or material shape, often called *'manifesting'*.

Working through the disturbances and imbalances that cause loss of sleep may prompt an exploration of the seven chakra areas. This can be a great tool for a client's self-exploration and you can assist with this process through offering practices that help to balance the areas that she (with your gentle assistance) identifies as needing support.

Below is a basic description according to the system as set out by Anodea Judith (1987) with some general correspondences between the various aspects of ourselves; we will consider how they relate to sleep. By our nature, we have some innate strengths and some areas of ourselves that we don't readily express. These may be under-developed, they may not have been reinforced, or we may have been told or have learnt through others' reactions that those parts of ourselves were not OK to express. Working through the chakra system offers us a way to identify what's over-developed (excessive) and what's under-developed (deficient), and to bring balance over time.

Strengths and Needs: 'Excess and Deficiency' within Each of the Chakras

The chakra system is a relatively simple way of understanding ourselves and our clients or students holistically. It takes the judgement out of looking at ourselves and others, and sees where we have 'strengths' in each area or where we have needs. In each area listed below, the aspect of ourselves may be over-done and become excessive or in each area we may be under-powered or lacking, resulting in a need or a deficiency. This type of understanding forms a non-judgemental, practical basis for a therapeutic programme.

The Chakras in Brief

CHAKRA ONE: MULADHARA – EARTH, PHYSICAL IDENTITY, SELF-PRESERVATION, SAFETY, SURVIVAL

Located at the base of the spine, this chakra forms our foundation. It corresponds to the element earth, and is related to structure, stability and survival. This relates to our sense of safety, and ability to be 'here' and to feel 'grounded'. Our sense of being present in the physical body relates to this. Imbalances in this area can be caused by feelings of danger or physical threat which can come from trauma or the experience of violence, or lack of resources to meet one's basic needs for food, shelter or money. When this area is 'deficient' it can mean that the person becomes either totally 'ungrounded' – becoming too thin or starving oneself – or over-compensating by hoarding, being greedy about money or over-eating.

CHAKRA TWO: SVADHISTHANA – WATER, EMOTIONAL IDENTITY, ORIENTED TO SELF-GRATIFICATION

The second chakra, located in the abdomen, lower back and sexual organs, is related to the element water, and to emotions, eros, polarity and sexuality. It represents our connection to others through feeling, desire, sensation and movement. Ideally this chakra represents the qualities of fluidity and grace, depth of feeling, sexual/sensual fulfilment and the ability to accept change. Some understandings of the chakra system relate eros to the power to create, as when two human beings reproduce and make another life. When this aspect is out of balance, a person may become too emotional and distressed, or suppress emotions to the point that they are expressed only in unconscious destructive acting out. Too much activity in the second chakra may be expressed as over-sexualization or co-dependency, both of which give an excess of energy to others, at the expense of one's own integrity, or can be expressed as a sexual or emotional form of anorexia, shutting down intimacy and sexuality. Without healthy expression of sensuality in relationship according to a person's needs, unnecessary tension and feelings of longing, loneliness or a lack of 'juiciness' in life can leave life feeling colourless.

CHAKRA THREE: MANIPURA – FIRE, EGO IDENTITY, ORIENTED TO SELF-DEFINITION

This chakra is known as the power chakra, located in the solar plexus. It relates to our sense of personal power, will and autonomy. It is located in the area of the stomach, and relates to our digestive fire, which is required for us to translate food into fuel for the 'fire' of doing things and accomplishing in life. When we are healthy in this area, we have a sense of 'get-up-and-go' or a 'fire in our belly' which connotes energy, effectiveness, spontaneity and non-dominating power. This is also located in the area of the adrenal glands, which secrete the stress hormones needed to spring into action. When they are over-activated we can experience 'burnout' and lethargy associated with having expended too much of our energy for too long. When we lack third chakra presence, we may be under-active in taking control of situations in our lives, and cede our will to others, asking them to take responsibility for us. If we are constantly in stress-mode, over-doing, this breaks our capacity to relax, while if we don't activate enough, this can mean we don't work up the homeostatic drive towards sleep.

CHAKRA FOUR: ANAHATA AIR – SOCIAL IDENTITY, ORIENTED TO SELF-ACCEPTANCE AND COMPASSION

This is called the heart chakra and is the midpoint of the seven-chakra system. It is related to love, and is seen as the integrator of opposites in the psyche: mind and body, masculine and feminine, persona and shadow, separateness and unity. A healthy fourth chakra allows us to love deeply, feel compassion, and have a deep sense of peace and centredness. It is located in the area of the heart and lungs – where the heartbeat and breath are the pulsations that sustain life. When we are afraid, our heart rate accelerates, our breathing speeds up, and we tighten up, constricting the chest in protection and shutting down the open-hearted quality we may feel when we are safe and loved. We tend to sleep poorly or over-sleep when we are broken-hearted, disconnected from love, are fearful, are not compassionate within ourselves, feel a lack of compassion or love from others, at times in the form of loneliness, or we may have loved and lost and are experiencing grief, or can't breathe easily for fear. All of these imbalances in the physical and energetic heart areas can lead to sleepless nights.

CHAKRA FIVE: VISHUDDHA – SOUND, CREATIVE IDENTITY, ORIENTED TO SELF-EXPRESSION

This is the chakra located in the throat and is thus related to communication and the expression of our creativity. Here we experience the world symbolically through vibration, such as the vibration of sound as it takes shape in language and in music. Imbalances in this area may relate to our communication with others – when we don't or can't communicate skilfully to meet our needs and negotiate meeting the needs of others, we can end up exhausted, depleted or resentful, which can cause us to lose sleep. When we speak in ways that create conflict within ourselves and in our lives, this can lead to sleepless nights. The throat area also encompasses the thyroid and parathyroid, which have important functions in our daily energy and in the regulation of sleep. When the thyroid is under-active (hypothyroid) we can become sluggish, needing too much sleep for not enough real rest. When it is over-active (hyperthyroid) we can become agitated, always 'on' and find it hard to rest, resulting in a sense of exhausted burnout related to the adrenal burnout mentioned in relationship to the third chakra.

CHAKRA SIX: AJNA – LIGHT, ARCHETYPAL IDENTITY, SELF-REFLECTION, INSIGHT AND CLEAR VISION

This is known as the brow chakra or third eye centre, and relates to the centre of the skull, right behind and in the centre of the two eyes, which corresponds with the pineal gland. It is related to seeing, both physically and in terms of intuitive understanding, and a balance of intellect with insight. When healthy it allows us to see clearly – in effect, letting us 'see the big picture'. When we lose perspective, and fail to see the long term, become narrow-minded or have an over-active mind fixated on stresses and concerns to the exclusion of calming and balancing forces, we can lose sleep or find getting to sleep difficult.

CHAKRA SEVEN: SAHASRARA – THOUGHT, CONNECTION
TO LIFE-FORCE AND SPIRITUAL UNDERSTANDING

The crown chakra relates to consciousness as 'pure awareness' and our connection to the greater matrices of life, to the mysterious connection to the life force that unites all beings. Developing this chakra brings us a broader perspective on our lives, a place that the poet Mary Oliver calls, in her poem 'Wild Geese' (2004), 'the family of things', and carries a sense of trust that comes from the sense of our smallness in that family of things, as well as our connection within it. When we don't have this understanding, lack a sense of spiritual connection (whether related to or completely unrelated to religion) and lack wonder and awe, life can seem dry, pointless and listless, and existential questions can keep us awake at night.

Distribution of Energy Among the Chakras

The energy in our body–mind system can be directed (marshalled and channelled) or it can be dissipated. The chakra system can serve as a guide that helps us to understand psychosomatic imbalances. We can see areas where energy/life force is said to be concentrated, over-active, stifled, flowing freely or 'leaky'. This relates to circulation and development in the physical structures of the body, and on a more subtle level the mental, emotional, psychological and spiritual aspects of ourselves.

If we operate on the understanding that we have a limited amount of energy each day, then energy spent in one area means that we have less energy to expend in the other areas of our lives. One metaphor used by Carolyn Myss (1997), who writes on the chakra system, is that it's as though we awake with £100 worth of energy every day to spend in any area of our lives. When we sleep we recharge the bank with 100 per cent of our daily energy allowance. If you were to spend £90 of your currency today to meet survival needs – seeking shelter or work or securing food – because you didn't have a place to live or enough food to eat, attention to the first chakra concerns of safety and security would leave you with only 10 per cent of your currency left to spend on other areas of life such as cultivating loving relationships (fourth chakra), spirituality (seventh chakra), etc.

If you were experiencing a bereavement, you might experience this as strong raw emotions of grief and sadness. The emotion-centre (second chakra) and heart might take 80 per cent of your energy on certain days, leaving only 20 per cent to be distributed to thinking/planning (sixth chakra) survival needs (first chakra) or getting work done (third chakra). Another person in the same situation might suppress feelings of grief, being, at least for a time, unable to cry or feel sadness, energetically shutting down the area related to the second chakra, and diverting attention and energy to 'doing things' (third chakra) or to tending to other people's emotional needs (fourth chakra).

Energy Within or Outside the System

In restoring balance to each of the chakra-related areas, and to rebalancing among them, a therapeutic programme involves practices that tend to all the areas. Many of my clients with insomnia spend a great deal of their time focusing on others, either as parents or carers, or at work devote tremendous resources of time and energy to their professional or occupational responsibilities. When all the attention in one's life force is directed towards serving others or towards an external pursuit, there is little left for maintaining balance within oneself, and our health and wellbeing can suffer from this lack of attention. The classic example of self-care is given when you board an aeroplane: the safety instructions always state that, in an emergency situation, you must place the oxygen mask on your own mouth and nose first, before assisting anyone else. You're no use to anyone if you can't breathe.

'Letting Go': The Power of Limitation, Endings and Finality

We can come to see ourselves as part of a greater spiritual context, and find a sense of integration and balance over time. Our daily concerns may be very real and pressing, but we realize that we are not ultimately 'in control' and that the worst that can happen is that we experience suffering or that we die. Many spiritual traditions deal directly with the difference between pain, which is inevitable, and suffering, which occurs when we fear pain, dwell on past pain, or presage pain in the future. The added suffering, with practice, can be recognized, and we may recognize it as unnecessary. The spiritual traditions deal directly with our fear of death and the finitude of endings, instead of dancing around the point. This, in my clinical experience, is very present for those who find it difficult to release into sleep. There is often a deep, existential, underlying fear that things won't be OK, and that we need to hold on 'for dear life' in some fundamental way. Because we are still, unprotected and not alert to our surroundings, we can't defend ourselves against threat – in a very real sense we are vulnerable to attack, even death. In ancient myths, when kings and gods fell asleep, it was then that their kingdoms and domains were vulnerable to attack. The myth states that, while Samson slept, Delilah cut his long flowing hair, and the source of his strength was stolen from him. The dream worlds brought promise and peril alike. They are not states of command and control – and anything can happen. The more fearful we are – consciously or unconsciously – of what we cannot fathom and cannot control, the less likely we are to sleep.

When there is trust in nature – or a force bigger than ourselves – that all will go on in its way, a sense of relaxation and release becomes possible. This is not to say that those who are 'spiritual' or who are happy and well adjusted will never fall ill or experience physical problems, nor is it to say that a person must be a 'spiritual person' to sleep well or be healthy. In fact, some of the pursuits undertaken by those on what may be called a spiritual path towards 'awakening' are *known* to keep you awake – to literally wake you up by stirring up the whole body–mind system to create transformation. However, if we are not functioning well in life, and are finding the colour drained out of every day because rest and sleep are eluding us, then something is calling out to us for attention. We may be called to awaken, to put life into a bigger perspective, and live each day fully.

Finding Meaning in a Fast-Moving World

It feels to many of my clients that insecurity and instability in work arrangements and relationships are rising. They speak about the new distractions – maybe even obligations – of the online world with its always-on nature, non-stop entertainment with streaming video services and potentially distressing news in a constant feed on tap day and night. Even if they are not part of the ever-growing population of people living on their own, it seems that loneliness and disconnection are themes that surface in their conversations. It may be that broader social, economic and technological trends affect our sense of security and safety and that, unless there is a conscious effort to stay slower and remain centred, many feel that life is lived faster than ever before.

> **Michelle** has finally ditched her sleeping pills. She does her yoga poses every night before bed, as a way to soothe her body and allow her mind to slow down. She notices the unresolved issues from the day as she slowly unravels the tension in her body. She finishes her yoga practice, writes down some notes for things she wants to resolve the next day, then closes her book, and puts it in the drawer of her bedside table, putting to bed her concerns. Initially, Michelle had resisted taking time to slow down during the day, but in the course of her sessions, she realized that she was living life as though it were one crisis after another, one external pressure after another. She scarcely gave herself time to breathe, much less rest or sleep. She has begun to find small moments to slow down, enjoy herself more and layer in rest when she is tired. She realized that taking time throughout the day gives her a sense of what her body needs, and she loves the luxurious quality of her bedtime ritual. When she doesn't have time for several poses, just a simple twist is enough to feel like a soothing balm for her body. She still finds meditation difficult, but using body-based techniques, she has started to unravel years of tension and, instead of hovering over her sheets, she settles more easily and sleeps more deeply.

It is possible that not-sleeping has a function or a purpose. For each individual, the signs of imbalance or distress show up differently. For an increasing number of us, a deeper unrest shows up as literal sleeplessness. Carl Jung (1973) spoke of the symptom as a symbol of something going on in our consciousness. He says that we may be 'too prone to regard a product [of the unconscious] that may actually be full of significance as a mere "symptom"' (para. 821). Something is either keeping us awake at night or is waking us up, and we might view this as a symbol of a deeper need or longing. Many of my 'insomniacs' find they have little time to themselves during the day and the time they get when they wake up in the middle of the night may be the only time they are not actually working or attending to family needs. This may be the 'soul's' way of taking personal time, quiet reflective time, as disturbing as this is to the daily habits.

My own insomnia called on me to learn about how to balance and soothe my body, manage my energy more carefully, come to know and work with my mind, listen to my emotions compassionately and put my life into a larger spiritual context. In peeling back these layers, bit by bit my sleep has become a litmus-test for what is going on in my life, and a move towards greater happiness and balance shows up as richer, more enjoyable and easier sleep. And when my sleep is disturbed, I know that something is amiss, and I can work to resolve what is troubling me.

Each of the clients whose stories you have heard in this book has been on a journey that we might call, in some way, spiritual. They have undertaken practices that have brought relief, communication and, ultimately, transformation.

> **Gary** came to yoga therapy because he had a form of depression combined with extreme lethargy, unrestful sleep and morning sluggishness. It wasn't long before his daughter shared sleep problems with her dad: she took longer and longer to fall asleep, and became increasingly groggy as she struggled to get ready for school. Gary began psychotherapy and added cycling and running back into his routine, along with morning yoga poses that got his circulation going, and added meditation into his day. This began a set of positive changes that helped him to address what was weighing him down. He began to feel more receptive to job recruiters, and eventually to taking on a new job that was more energizing. With a renewed sense of purpose, he felt happier, more connected with his family and slept more easily. As Gary became more lighthearted, he noticed a general change in his family – his daughter began sleeping through the night and waking up refreshed.

What we experience in our own healing, we pass along to those around us. When people look after themselves well – beyond personal grooming and luxuries to the deeper longings – they often sleep better. As Dr Jim Horne, whom I mentioned in the Introduction, noted, 'When people are happier they sleep better.' This creates a virtuous cycle. It's both a pleasure and an honour to help people create this kind of self-care.

Healing Work as a Meaningful – Even Sacred – Service

In helping other people sleep, therapists, doctors, yoga teachers and body workers can become *sleuths*, helping to sniff out where the disturbance may originate. We also become *teachers and coaches*, imparting new information and techniques to help soothe, calm and rest when needed, and to mobilize energy when needed. We also take on the role that *parents* do with babies, helping our charges learn to self-soothe, offering explicit techniques, but also, ideally, we show them something in the calmness with which we receive them. We can help our clients to know that it is safe to let go and be 'held' in the arms of sleep. We also become expert *interpreters* in that we help them to understand what the tension, restlessness and sleeplessness are telling them about their lives. We can open up questions and invite our clients to find the answers for themselves. By moving through the layers in this programme, you're giving guidance to a person, to acknowledge different parts of themselves, to become aware of balance or imbalance and to use the imbalances as cues to make change.

Helping and healing ourselves and others is a way to give life meaning. When I was a little girl, I was given a simple spiritual teaching by my parents: 'Leave it better than you found it.' I took this to mean: 'Contribute positively to the world around you, in the way that you can.' I was also taught that if you have your health, then everything else is easier, so this is a fundamental part of contributing to the world, rather than a luxury. When I encountered crushing insomnia, I knew I didn't want a life of pill-popping pathology, and that there had to be a better way. So I set out to find it. The result is here, in these pages.

I was also taught that if you give and receive love, in this life, it will be a well-lived life, full of the riches that count most. You may be very in touch with a calling in life to help others, or you may have stumbled into it and are now considering this aspect to your professional practice. The techniques and approaches in this book offer you a way to enhance your own wellbeing, as well as offering something of value to others' lives.

When you start using the practices in this book, you will learn or refine your tools, and develop your skills. Asana practices help you to tune into the tension and release in the body that give us the capacity to feel what's needed for good sleep and vibrant days. When you practise the techniques in this book, you learn how to move to feel either relaxed and more grounded for sleep, or to activate the body at the right times of day so that it can build up the drive to sleep. When you pay attention to the physical sensations in your own body, you will become more aware of what is happening in your clients and students, and be able to see and feel what is needed in working with them more clearly. When you practise the breathing exercises (pranayama) and know them in your own body, can feel their effects on your own circulation, heartbeat and mental state, you will be a better guide for others, as you will understand the shifts you feel in yourself and be better able to sense when your clients have 'got it'. The same goes for the mental and emotional tools – when you have a practice of meditation, you're not just saying words to your clients, but can convey the richness of what it means to drop into a relaxed, conscious state. People who meditate have a sense of it, and convey this sense in how they talk about it, teach it and pass it on. Similarly, having contact with emotions – with compassion internally – means we are more compassionate and accepting of our clients, more patient when needed, more boundaried when needed. We become more equanimous by not pushing away the difficult things, and this gives permission to those around us to be themselves, which is inherently calming. And when we see what we do to help others as a way to serve, to give life meaning and to simply take part in the human endeavour, then we become better at it, less ego-driven, and ultimately more effective in the process of healing.

When you practise, you become a more subtle healer. After using the tools for some time yourself, observing your responses, and using them with your clients for some time, watching how they respond to the practices, you will become so skilful in using them that you can become more intuitive in what you give and when you give it. If you work with these tools, like any craftsperson or artisan, your way of using the tools and skills will become more easeful and masterful – and you can teach and guide others with great confidence, compassion and care.

Blessing between Teacher and Student

ॐ सह नाववतु ।

सह नौ भुनक्तु ।

सह वीर्यं करवावहै ।

तेजस्वि नावधीतमस्तु मा विद्विषावहै ।

ॐ शान्तिः शान्तिः शान्तिः ॥

Om Saha Naav[au]-Avatu |

Saha Nau Bhunaktu |

Saha Viiryam Karavaavahai |

Tejasvi Naav[au]-Adhiitam-Astu Maa Vidvissaavahai |

Om Shaantih Shaantih Shaantih | |

Meaning

Om, May God Protect Us Both (the Teacher and the Student) (during the journey of awakening our Knowledge),

May God Nourish Us Both (with that spring of Knowledge which nourishes life when awakened),

May We Work Together with Energy and Vigour (cleansing ourselves with that flow of energy for the Knowledge to manifest),

May Our Study be Enlightening (taking us towards the true Essence underlying everything), and Not Giving Rise to Hostility (by constricting the understanding of the Essence in a particular manifestation only),

Om, Peace, Peace, Peace (be there in the three levels – Adhidaivika, Adhibhautika and Adhyatmika).

References

Arnaud, M.J. (1987) 'The pharmacology of caffeine.' *Progress in Drug Research/ Fortschritte Der Arzneimittelforschung/Progrès Des Recherches Pharmaceutiques 31*, 273–313. doi:10.1007/978-3-0348-9289-6_9

Benson, H. and Klipper, M.Z. (2001) *The Relaxation Response*. New York: Quill.

Brown, B. (2010) *TED Talk: The Power of Vulnerability*. Accessed on 18/10/2018 at www.ted.com/talks/brene_brown_on_vulnerability.

Brown, R.R. and Gerbarg, P.L. (2012) *The Healing Power of the Breath: Simple Techniques to Reduce Stress and Anxiety, Enhance Concentration, and Balance Your Emotions*. Boston: Shambhala.

Buysse, D.J. (2013) 'Insomnia.' *Journal of the American Medical Association 309*, 7, 706–716.

Chang, A., Aeschbach, D., Duffy, J.F. and Czeisler, C.A. (2014) 'Evening use of light-emitting eReaders negatively affects sleep, circadian timing, and next-morning alertness.' *Proceedings of the National Academy of Sciences 112*, 4, 1232–1237. doi:10.1073/pnas.1418490112

Dreams (2016) *The 2016 UK Sleep Survey Results*. Accessed on 14/9/2018 at www.dreams.co.uk/sleep-matters-club/sleep-survey-uk-2016.

Emerson, D. (2015) *Trauma-Sensitive Yoga in Therapy: Bringing the Body into Treatment*. New York: W.W. Norton & Company.

Feuerstein, G. (n.d.) *Yoga and Yoga Therapy*. Accessed on 20/7/2018 at www.iayt. org/?page=YogaAndYogaTherapy.

Feuerstein, G. (2011) *The Path of Yoga: An Essential Guide to Its Principles and Practices*. Boston: Shambhala.

Feuerstein, G. (2014) *The Psychology of Yoga: Integrating Eastern and Western Approaches for Understanding the Mind*. Boston: Shambhala.

Frawley, D. (2000) *Ayurvedic Healing: A Comprehensive Guide*. Twin Lakes, WI: Lotus Press.

Frawley, D. (2005) *Ayurveda and the Mind: The Healing of Consciousness*. Delhi: Motilal Banarsidass.

Frawley, D. (2013) *Yoga and Ayurveda: Self-Healing and Self-Realization*. Delhi: Motilal Banarsidass.

Frawley, D., Ranade, S. and Lele, A. (2003) *Ayurveda and Marma Therapy: Energy Points in Yogic Healing*. Twin Lakes, WI: Lotus Press.

Gerbarg, P. and Brown, R. (2005) 'Sudarshan Kriya yogic breathing in the treatment of stress, anxiety, and depression: Part I – Neurophysiologic model.' *The Journal of Alternative and Complementary Medicine 11*, 1, 189–201.

Hanh, T.N. (2016) *How to Love.* London: Rider.

Härle, D. (2017) *Trauma-Sensitive Yoga.* London: Singing Dragon.

Hauri, P. and Linde, S.M. (1996) *No More Sleepless Nights.* New York: Wiley.

Havens, C.M., Grandner, M.A., Youngstedt, S.D., Pandey, A. and Parthasarathy, S. (2017) 'International variability in the prevalence of insomnia and use of sleep-promoting medications, supplements and other substances.' *Sleep 40* (Suppl 1), A117–A118.

Herman, J.L. (1992) *Trauma and Recovery.* New York: Basic Books.

Horne, J. (2007) *Sleepfaring: A Journey Through the Science of Sleep.* Oxford: Oxford University Press.

Horne, J. (2016) *Sleeplessness: Assessing Sleep Need in Society Today.* Cham: Palgrave Macmillan.

Iyengar, B.K.S. (1995) *Light on Yoga.* London: Schocken Books.

Judith, A. (1987) *Wheels of Life: A User's Guide to the Chakra System.* St. Paul, MN: Llewellyn Publications.

Jung, C.G. (1973) 'Psychological Types.' In *Collected Works of C.G. Jung: The First Complete English Edition of the Works of C.G. Jung.* London: Routledge.

Karl, L. (2012) 'Compassionate presence: teaching Trauma-Sensitive Yoga.' *Yoga Therapy Today*, September, 20–22. Accessed on 20/7/2018 at https://mettayoga.files.wordpress.com/2011/10/ytt-summer-insight.pdf.

Khalsa, S.B. with Gould, J. (2012) *Your Brain on Yoga: A Harvard Health Book.* Harvard University. Accessed on 14/5/2018 at www.harvardhealthbooks.org/wp-content/uploads/2013/03/YourBrainOnYogaSampleChapter.pdf.

Koay, J. (2012) *Science & Philosophy of Teaching Yoga & Yoga Therapy.* Sun Yoga Press.

Lad, V. (2007) *Textbook of Ayurveda: A Complete Guide to Clinical Assessment* (Volume 2). Albuquerque: Ayurvedic Press. UK edition.

Lasater, J. (2011) *Relax and Renew: Restful Yoga for Stressful Times.* Berkeley, CA: Rodmell Press.

Levine, P.A. (1997) *Waking the Tiger: Healing Trauma.* Berkeley, CA: North Atlantic Books.

Levine, P.A. (2008) *Healing Trauma: A Pioneering Program for Restoring the Wisdom of Your Body.* Boulder, CO: Sounds True.

Levine, P.A. (2010) *In an Unspoken Voice: How the Body Releases Trauma and Restores Goodness.* Berkeley: North Atlantic Books.

Mariposa, B. (2018) *Mindfulness Playbook: How to Bring Calm and Happiness into Your Daily Life.* London: Hodder & Stoughton.

Mason, H. (2017) 'Mechanisms of pranayama: how respiratory physiology can refine your teaching.' *Yoga Therapy Today*, Spring.

Mason, H. and Birch, K. (eds) (2018) *Yoga for Mental Health.* Edinburgh: Handspring Publishing.

Murphy, P.J. and Campbell, S.S. (1997) 'Nighttime drop in body temperature: a physiological trigger for sleep onset?' *Sleep 20*, 7, 505–511. doi:10.1093/sleep/20.7.505

Myss, C.M. (1997) *Anatomy of the Spirit: The Seven Stages of Power and Healing.* Sydney: Bantam Books.

National Sleep Foundation (n.d.) *Sleep Diary.* Accessed on 20/7/2018 at https://sleepfoundation.org/sites/default/files/SleepDiaryv6.pdf.

Olivelle, P. (1998) *Upaniṣads.* Oxford: Oxford University Press.

Oliver, M. (2004) *Wild Geese: Selected Poems.* Tarset: Bloodaxe.

Rogers, C.R. (1961) *On Becoming a Person: A Therapist's View of Psychotherapy.* Boston: Houghton Mifflin.

Rosenberg, M. (2003) *Nonviolent Communication: A Language of Life.* Encinitas, CA: Puddle Dancer Press.

Roth, T., Coulouvrat, C., Hajak, G., Lakoma, M.D. *et al.* (2011) 'Prevalence and perceived health associated with insomnia based on DSM-IV-TR; International Statistical Classification of Diseases and Related Health Problems, Tenth Revision; and Research Diagnostic Criteria/International Classification of Sleep Disorders, Second Edition criteria: results from the America Insomnia Survey.' *Biological Psychiatry 69*, 6, 592–600.

Shannahoff-Khalsa, D. (2006) *Kundalini Yoga Meditation: Techniques Specific for Psychiatric Disorders, Couples Therapy, and Personal Growth.* New York: Norton.

Shearer, A. (trans. and ed.) (2002) *The Yoga Sutras of Patanjali.* New York: Bell Tower.

Sleep Council (2017) *Great British Bedtime Report.* Accessed on 14/9/2018 at https://sleepcouncil.org.uk/wp-content/uploads/2018/04/The-Great-British-Bedtime-Report-2017.pdf.

St-Onge, M., Mikic, A. and Pietrolungo, C.E. (2016) 'Effects of diet on sleep quality.' *Advances in Nutrition 7*, 5, 938–949. doi:10.3945/an.116.012336

Stiles, M. (2010) *Ayurvedic Yoga Therapy.* Twin Lakes, WI: Lotus Press.

Stiles, M. (2013) *Structural Yoga Therapy: Adapting to the Individual.* San Francisco, CA: Weiser Books.

Streeter, C., Gerbarg, P. and Saper, R. (2012) 'Yoga therapy associated with increased brain GABA levels and decreased depressive symptoms in subjects with major depressive disorder: a pilot study.' *BMC Complementary and Alternative Medicine 12*, Suppl 1, P31. doi:10.1186/1472-6882-12-S1-P31

Weintraub, A. (2004) *Yoga for Depression.* New York: Broadway Books.

Wong, C.K., Marshall, N.S., Grunstein, R.R., Hibbs, D.E. *et al.* (2016) 'Spontaneous adverse event reports associated with zolpidem.' *Research in Social and Administrative Pharmacy 12*, 5, e24. doi:10.1016/j.sapharm.2016.05.062

Wong, C.K., Marshall, N.S., Grunstein, R.R., Ho, S.S. *et al.* (2017) 'Spontaneous adverse event reports associated with zolpidem in the United States 2003–2012.' *Journal of Clinical Sleep Medicine 13*, 2, 223–234. doi:10.5664/jcsm.6452

About the Author

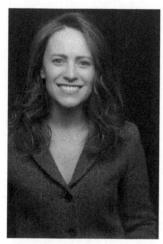

Photo: Claire Newman-Williams

Lisa Sanfilippo is a senior yoga teacher, psychotherapist, writer/researcher and yoga therapy for insomnia expert.

With over 20 years of experience, and having herself overcome crippling insomnia, today Lisa's programmes help thousands of others to sleep better through practical yoga and a body–mind wellness system. Her work is road-tested, evidence-based and practical. She has worked with athletes, captains of industry, actors, stressed-out parents, older adults and children using her methods, with great success.

Lisa holds a BSc from Brown University and an MSc from the London School of Economics, and trained as a psychotherapist at the Centre for Counselling and Psychotherapy Education in London, where she completed MA research into the intersections of yoga and transpersonal psychotherapy in conjunction with Northampton University. She is a Senior Teacher and Teacher Trainer at Triyoga UK, a long-standing teacher at The Life Centre, an IAYT-registered Yoga Therapist, and has served as an adjunct teacher at the Minded Institute. With Yogacampus' yoga therapy Diploma programme she offers both training modules and continuing professional development.

Lisa has created the Sleep Recovery Yoga online course (www.sleeprecoveryyoga.com) and offers teacher training in her methods. She also offers training to corporations, medical practices and others wishing to incorporate the principles of yoga therapy for sleep and insomnia into their clinical work, or to help employees/clients to improve rest, sleep performance and wellbeing.

Index